Becoming Multiculturally Responsible on Campus

FROM AWARENESS TO ACTION

Max Parker
University of Florida

Jennifer Sager

Lahaska Press
Houghton Mifflin Company
Boston   New York

To Mr. Mark A. Parker, Jr. and Mrs. Bobbie M. Parker-Dailey, my older brother and sister, who inspired, supported, and taught me the real meaning of responsibility.

—WMP

To Veronica,

So that multicultural responsibility becomes an expected trait in our society by the time you attend college.

—JBS

Publisher, Lahaska Press: Barry Fetterolf
Senior Editor, Lahaska Press: Mary Falcon
Senior Marketing Manager, Lahaska Press: Barbara LeBuhn
Senior Project Editor: Margaret Park Bridges
Cover Design Manager: Anne S. Katzeff
Senior Composition Buyer: Chuck Dutton
New Title Project Manager: Susan Brooks-Peltier
Editorial Assistant: Evangeline Bermas

Cover Image: © Images.com / CORBIS / Jim Frazier

For instructors who want more information about Lahaska Press books and teaching aids, contact the Houghton Mifflin Faculty Services Center at
   Tel: 800-733-1717, x4034
   Fax: 800-733-1810
Or visit us on the Web at **www.lahaskapress.com**.

Lahaska Press, established as an imprint of Houghton Mifflin Company in 1999, is dedicated to publishing textbooks and instructional media for counseling and the helping professions. Its editorial offices are located in the small town of Lahaska, Pennsylvania. *Lahaska* is a Native American Lenape word meaning "source of much writing."

Printed in the U.S.A.

Library of Congress Control Number: 2007926454

Instructor's examination copy
   ISBN-10: 0-618-73350-7
   ISBN-13: 978-0-618-73350-7

For orders, use student text ISBNs
   ISBN-10: 0-618-49294-1
   ISBN-13: 978-0-618-49294-7

123456789-EB-11 10 09 08 07

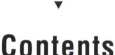

Contents

CHAPTER 3

Recognizing and Overcoming Privilege   57

CHAPTER 4

Racial, Ethnic, Cultural, and Gender Variables in the Classroom   80

Preface

This book is new and different from other books designed to sensitize college students to diversity issues on campus. Unlike many other books that usually stop at the consciousness-raising level regarding cultural, racial, gender, sexual orientation, socioeconomic, and other differences, we have raised the ante by challenging students to become more responsible or accountable in their responses or actions in multicultural situations. It has been our observation that too many college students have learned the politically correct language to convince others that they are culturally sensitive, but their actions do not match their words. We have written this book to not only challenge students but to support them as they strive to become multiculturally responsible persons (MRPs). We have carefully selected and used examples and experiences reflective of all areas of campus life throughout this book to achieve this goal. In cases where scenarios or examples are used, fictitious names are used and experiences are revised to protect confidentiality.

Although these writers have somewhat different philosophies on methods of diversity training, they compliment one another very well in their writing together in this book. Max tends to be more laid back while Jennifer tends to be more forthright. This two-headed combination of philosophies, which is integrated throughout this book, is essential for achieving the delicate balance of pushing hard and pushing softly to move college students toward personal growth in general and toward becoming multiculturally responsible in particular.

As such, this book is organized into seven chapters that encourage multicultural responsibility in various aspects of college life. We believe that this organization allows for college students to more personally relate to the complex issues of race, ethnicity, and culture and will encourage continued dialogue with friends and classmates. In Chapter 1 we introduce the basics of multicultural responsibility. Readers will take several informal assessments and begin to understand the roadblocks to multicultural responsibility. In Chapter 2 there is an explanation of how people develop a racial, ethnic, and cultural identity. We present various identity models and action plans designed to facilitate advancement in identity stages. In Chapter 3 we address the complex issues of privilege against the backdrop of the college experience. Different types of privilege, including those not typically addressed such as gender identity, ability, and economic privilege, are explored. In Chapter 4 we focus on multicultural issues in the classroom, such as classroom expectation, presentation of diversity material in lectures and textbooks, and communicating with instructors. In Chapter 5 we present information on variables within housing and extracurricular activities. This chapter focuses on the concept that much of college learning occurs outside the classroom with peers. Although not all colleges will have the same housing options and extracurricular activities, we attempt to present a variety of experiences that capture the majority of out-of-classroom diversity learning. In Chapter 6 we address the interaction of multiculturalism and intimate relationships. We examine advanced gender issues, interracial friendships and dating, same-sex dating, and sexual harassment. Chapter 7 is our conclusion and final suggestions about how to become multiculturally responsible.

Throughout this book you will find exercises to increase your interest in becoming more multiculturally responsible. *Diversity definitions* consist of a list of frequently used terms and terms that are often confusing to readers. *Reflection* exercises encourage readers to think about their own lives while thinking about their surroundings. These exercises can often be completed through contemplation or journal writing. Other more challenging exercises encourage people to move beyond the ponder stage and into personal action or discussions with other people. We hope that through these exercises you will be able to learn and instructors will be able to guide you on the course of multicultural responsibility.

We—Woodrow M. Parker, an African-American man, and Jennifer Sager, a Jewish-American woman—have both struggled with diversity issues throughout our personal and professional lives. I (Dr. Parker) received my Ph.D. in Counselor Education from the University of Florida in 1975. Over the past 25 years I have been involved in teaching, counseling, and training with the major focus on multicultural and diversity issues. I have written several books and have authored and co-authored more than 40 articles in refereed journals on the subject of multiculturalism. I (Dr. Sager) received my Ph.D. in Counseling Psychology from The Pennsylvania State University in 2005 and enjoyed being a staff member of the University of Florida's Counseling Center for seven years. Most recently, I have been working in private practice and in the area of consultation. I have presented on the national and state level, as well as published, on a variety of topics, including how the college experience differs based on race, sexual orientation, and transgender identity.

It is our hope that our combined experience in teaching multiculturalism— and the personal strengths we have gained from confronting the positives and negatives of the diversity of American society on our own lives—will help college students become multiculturally responsible through the variety of creative, thought provoking, and personally challenging experiences addressed in this book.

ACKNOWLEDGMENTS

We owe a debt of gratitude to many people who have contributed to this book. First, we want to thank Dr. Allen Ivey for his creative guidance and suggestions that he provided in the early stages of development of this book. As a scholar who has written many books on multiculturalism, his advice was most valuable. The manuscript was made much stronger with salient input from the Division of Student Affairs of Santa Fe Community College. In particular, we want to thank Dr. Portia Taylor, Vice President for Student Affairs; Dr. Mardell Coleman, Director of the Counseling Center; Ms. Elizabeth O'Reggio, Director of the Office of Diversity; and Dr. W. Dontray Rollins, Specialist, Office of Diversity. It was through their examples that a greater understanding of the multicultural issues in the community college system was provided.

We are grateful to work with so many talented and culturally sensitive people at the University of Florida. In particular, we would like to thank Dr. Mary Kay Schneider, Associate Dean of Students, and Ms. Ann Ho-Becks, Assistant Dean and Director of New Student Programs, who challenged us to expand our definition of multiculturalism to be more inclusive of the wide range of diversity in our diverse world. The support of our colleagues from the University of Florida Counseling Center and Student Mental Health was also invaluable.

Several people are responsible for helping us create a close friendship. We want to thank Rachel Horde for encouraging us to co-teach the multi-cultural counseling course, Dr. Angela Ferguson for solidifying our relationship, and Dr. LaTrelle Jackson for encouraging us to write this book.

I, Jennifer, would like to thank several wonderful people who made it clear that White individuals can be race allies, especially when I doubted myself. In this regard, I want to express thanks and love to Dr. Beverly Vandiver, Dr. Angela Ferguson, Dr. LaTrelle Jackson, Dr. Anne Heath, Dr. Shari Robinson, Dr. Natasha Maynard-Pemba, and Dr. Carlos Hernandez. I would also like to thank my mom, Dawn Ross, and my father, Robert Sager, for teaching me to respect others and to cherish differences even though we might disagree about vocabulary, interracial dating, and "gay day" at Disney. You taught me to be headstrong and you were there for me when the world was not tolerant of this trait.

I, Max, want to thank my mother, Mrs. Nellie J. Parker, for cultivating within me through her life example, the strength to be a forgiving individual. No matter how much she was mistreated, she lived in peace because she had the strength to forgive herself and to forgive others. As a multicultural specialist, I have learned that there is no better way to manage race-related guilt than through the process of forgiveness. Again, thank you mother.

Several individuals shared their personal experiences and allowed us to use their voices to help others become multiculturally responsible. We are thankful to Tina Davis, Scott Cohen, Woodja Flanigan, Ed Crain, Charles Byrd, and Lauren Gustafson. We would like to thank the anonymous individuals who responded to our Internet survey and the instructors at colleges across the country who graciously provided helpful feedback as manuscript reviewers. Our book is fresh and reflective of current thought because of their input:

Elizabeth Coccia, Austin Community College

Tim Cook, Clark College

Jacqueline Elder, Triton College

Jacqueline Griswold, Holyoke Community College

Calvenea Malloy, Mesa Community College

Fritz G. Polite, University of Central Florida

Cheryl Rohrbaugh, Northern Virginia Community College

Walter Swett Jr., Quinsigamond Community College

We want to thank our spouses, Ms. Sylvia B. Parker and Mr. Chris Brown, for their meticulous word processing, grammatical corrections, patience, love, and support. In addition, we also want to thank Ms. Susan Brown at the Education Library for her passion in providing the wealth of resource materials.

We are grateful to Lahaska Press, a division of Houghton Mifflin, and especially our editor, Barry Fetterolf, for his support, encouragement, and dedication. His patience in our delayed deadlines was appreciated. Special appreciation goes to our developmental editor, Bruce Cantley, who deftly understood and respected our direction. Your clarity and focus helped strengthen our words, voice, and spirit.

Finally, we want to acknowledge that we are not the only creators of the many techniques and strategies used to foster multicultural responsibility. Many advocates of cultural diversity have emphasized the idea that we need to move from talk about multiculturalism to actions of multicultural responsibility. We are thankful for those contributors.

CHAPTER 1

▲▲▲
▼▼▼

Understanding Multicultural Responsibility

BEFORE YOU READ

1. What is your definition of the term *multiculturalism*? What experiences in your life have made you arrive at that definition? Have you taken courses in multiculturalism or learned about the term in other ways?

2. Do you consider yourself sensitive to matters of multiculturalism? In what ways have you demonstrated sensitivity to people different from yourself in your life? Are you equally sensitive to people from different races, genders, sexual orientations, religions, nationalities, and so forth? If so, how so? If not, in your opinion are some groups more deserving of sensitivity than others?

3. What are your definitions of the terms *race, ethnicity,* and *culture*? Do these terms all mean the same thing or are they distinct? Can they be distinct yet cross over each other in some ways?

4. What are your definitions of the terms *prejudice, discrimination*, and *stereotyping*? Do these terms all mean the same thing or are they distinct?

5. Think of the various multicultural groups that exist in the world and on campus and the terms they prefer to use to describe themselves and be described by others. What terms do you think are appropriate and what terms do you think are inappropriate? Why?

INTRODUCTION

Imagine this scenario: Students enrolled in a multicultural education course in college break into small groups. The instructor asks the students to discuss how they could be more multiculturally sensitive in a diverse classroom. One student, a Latina American, begins the conversation by saying that she is already multiculturally sensitive because of her Latin American ethnicity. She goes on to say that because she has experienced prejudice firsthand, she has a natural understanding of diversity issues. A White male classmate is afraid to disagree with the first student's comments, fearing that he will be dismissed because of his "whiteness" if he speaks up.

Is the Latina female inherently aware of diversity because of her ethnicity? Do her classroom comments express her multicultural sensitivity? Although it is likely

> **DEFINITION**
>
> *Multicultural sensitivity* involves being aware of different multicultural issues such as race, ethnicity, sexual orientation, and gender.

> **DEFINITION**
>
> *Multicultural responsibility* is the concept of being aware of multicultural differences and allowing this awareness to empower our interactions with other people.

> **DEFINITION**
>
> *Hispanic American* or *Latino/Latina American*? Deciding which of these terms to use is a complicated issue that often differs based on birthplace, family heritage, politics, preference, and other factors. To count in the national Census those individuals from a Spanish/Latin American heritage, the U.S. government created the term *Hispanic*, which includes individuals who differ greatly in terms of skin color, physical characteristics, religion, and fluency in Spanish. The terms *Latino* (for men) and *Latina* (for women) originated from the community itself and are often seen as less formal. Some people use the term *Hispanic American* to represent those individuals who immigrated from Spain and use the terms *Latino* and *Latina* to represent those individuals from Latin America. As such, a Colombian individual might feel comfortable using either the term *Hispanic* (because of the Spanish influence) or *Latino* (because of geography), but a Brazilian individual is more likely to use *Latino*, because the Portuguese (not Spain) colonized Brazil. Others prefer to use more specific terms. For example, people who are of Mexican origin and living in the United States may prefer the terms *Chicano* or *Chicana*. Because there is still not a consensus about which term is most appropriate, we will use the terms *Hispanic American* and *Latino/Latina American* interchangeably in this book.

that she has an advantage over other students because of her own experience with prejudice, her own ethnicity does not automatically make her an expert on diversity. At the same time, is the White student doing the right thing by deciding to keep quiet? Who is demonstrating more multicultural responsibility in this classroom situation? The Latina American female shuts down other students, shaming them into being quiet. The White male shuts down his own learning process for fear of being called prejudiced. As a result, neither of these students is exhibiting multicultural responsibility.

Unfortunately, the preceding potentially useful multicultural classroom exercise has ended up driving a wedge between these students, possibly scaring them away from further multicultural growth in college. As we will explore in this book, learning multicultural responsibility is a long and challenging task, which can be even more challenging when individuals assume that their experiences automatically make them experts on multiculturalism (or the opposite) and judge others as prejudiced. Learning multicultural responsibility is more meaningful when it involves a group of dedicated people who are mostly aware of their own diversity issues and are willing to explore these issues further.

MULTICULTURALLY RESPONSIBLE PARTICIPANT (MRP) ASSESSMENT EXERCISES

An important first step in increasing multicultural responsibility is the exploration of self-awareness. Through the two assessment exercises included in this section, we will examine your personal awareness, experiences with diversity, and the level of multicultural awareness or knowledge that you, the Multiculturally Responsible Participant (MRP) may have at this time.

> ### DEFINITION
>
> **Multiculturally Responsible Participant (MRP)** is our term for an individual who is interested both in learning how to involve himself or herself in personal multicultural exploration and in making personal and systematic changes in multicultural responses. In other words, you, the reader, have the opportunity and potential to become an MRP.

Personal Assessment Survey

The first assessment exercise is an eight-item, open-ended survey designed to help you to examine your personal feelings about, attitudes toward, and perceptions of people from other racial, ethnic, and cultural groups. This personal assessment survey is designed to help you, the MRP, think about or discuss with others how you feel about yourself as a member of a racial/ethnic/cultural group.

DEFINITIONS

Race, ethnicity, and *culture.* The terms *race, ethnicity*, and *culture* have multiple definitions and these definitions often overlap with one another. A geneticist's definition will often differ from an anthropologist's definition. We will use the most common definitions of each term, as defined here, for the remainder of this book. *Race* typically refers to the genetic, physical characteristics of a group that can be observed by other individuals, such as skin color and certain identifiable facial features. *Ethnicity* typically refers to the ancestry of a person and the religious and/or linguistic characteristics that come with ancestry; examples of ethnic groups would be Russians, New Zealand Maoris, Brazilians, and Jews (even though existing within many nationalities, Jews are often considered to be an ethnic group because of a shared religious faith and use of the Hebrew language in religious ceremonies). *Culture* typically refers to social characteristics shared within a particular population; for instance, Lesbian, Gay, Bisexual, and Transgender (LGBT) culture might include a shared knowledge of important historical moments in the groups' struggles for civil rights, or a mutual appreciation for a symbol that represents the LGBT community in a positive way, such as the rainbow flag.

Personal Assessment Survey (PAS)

(Adapted from Parker, Archer, & Scott, 1992)

DIRECTIONS: Answer each of the eight following questions by writing down your initial thoughts, reactions, and feelings (please give your immediate reaction rather than becoming too engaged in deep self-exploration). Then discuss your responses with another student and later with a small group. Finally, these items can be discussed with the whole class.

1. Identify your own racial/ethnic/cultural group (biracial, Native American, Asian American, Hispanic/Latino(a) American, African American, Lesbian/ Gay/Bisexual/Transgender (LGBT), European American, Jewish, etc.) and think about why you are proud to be a member of your group.

2. What do you remember from your childhood about the attitudes and feelings of other important people in your life (parents, close relatives, close friends, teachers, counselors, etc.) toward people from racial/ethnic/ cultural groups different from your own group? Can you remember any specific comments or phrases used by the people around you to describe other groups? Can you think of ways your attitudes and feelings toward racially/ethnically/culturally different people have been influenced by these people?

3. Identify and discuss ways that being a member of your racial/ethnic/ cultural group has been an advantage to you and ways that it has been a disadvantage to you.

4. Identify and discuss at least one way that your upbringing has influenced your outlook on life.

5. Identify and discuss briefly one situation involving racially/ethnically/culturally different individuals where you have felt or would feel most comfortable and one where you have felt or would feel most uncomfortable.

6. In which ways, if any, does being a member of your racial/ethnic/cultural group affect your relationship with racially/ethnically/culturally different individuals?

7. What generalizations do you believe racially/ethnically/culturally different individuals make about your racial/ethnic/cultural group?

8. Identify and discuss briefly at least one significant fact you would like racially/ethnically/culturally different individuals to know and understand about your racial/ethnic/cultural group.

To which of the above questions did you have the strongest reaction? Explain. Are there any personal changes you would like to make?

An important first step in becoming an MRP is to learn that everyone has a history that influences his or her beliefs, attitudes, and feelings. Knowledge and awareness of your own history will help you become more accepting and understanding of people from racial/ethnic/cultural groups different from your own. It is hoped that this self-assessment will not only cause changes in the way you think and feel, but will also "jump start" you toward specific action. More specifically, you can learn more about your own history by talking with immediate family members, relatives, and friends; by reading family histories; and by searching the Internet for information on your own racial/ethnic/cultural history. The process of learning more about your own heritage will help to build your own self-esteem, an important step toward becoming an MRP.

Multicultural Experience Inventory

This second assessment exercise is designed to help MRPs explore and become more aware of the extent of their early and current life experiences with diversity. The Multicultural Experience Inventory consists of 16 items written in a sentence completion format. The first eight items cover your early life experiences, and the last eight items (9–16) cover your current experiences with various ethnic/racial/cultural groups.

Multicultural Experience Inventory

(Adapted from Ramirez, 1991)

DIRECTIONS: Complete the following 16 items by circling one of the five racial/ethnic/cultural identity choices. Then respond to the five questions that follow the inventory.

a = Almost entirely my racial/ethnic/cultural group (Note: cultural groups include LGBT people and people with disabilities)

b = Mostly my racial/ethnic/cultural group with a few people from other groups

c = Mixed (my racial/ethnic/cultural group plus numerous people from other groups)

d = Mostly people from other racial/ethnic/cultural groups with a few people from my own group

e = Almost entirely people from other racial/ethnic/cultural groups

1. The racial/ethnic/cultural composition of the neighborhoods in which I grew up was   a   b   c   d   e.

2. My childhood friends who visited my home and related well to my parents were   a   b   c   d   e.

3. The teachers and counselors with whom I had the closest relationships growing up were   a   b   c   d   e.

4. The people who have most influenced me in my education have been a   b   c   d   e.

5. In high school, my close friends were   a   b   c   d   e.

6. The ethnic backgrounds of the people I have dated have been a   b   c   d   e.

7. In the jobs I have had, my close friends have been   a   b   c   d   e.

8. The people with whom I have established close, meaningful relationships have been   a   b   c   d   e.

9. At present, my close friends are   a   b   c   d   e.

10. My close friends at work are   a   b   c   d   e.

11. I enjoy going to gatherings at which the people are   a   b   c   d   e.

12. When I study or work on a project with others, I am usually with persons who are   a   b   c   d   e.

13. When I am involved in group discussions in which I am expected to participate, I prefer a group of people who are   a   b   c   d   e.

14. I am active in organizations or social groups in which the majority of members are   a   b   c   d   e.

15. When I am with my friends, I usually attend functions where the people are   a   b   c   d   e.

16. When I discuss personal problems or issues, I discuss them with people who are   a   b   c   d   e.

DIRECTIONS: Answer each question individually and join a small group for further discussion.

1. What impressed you most about your multicultural experience? Were there any surprises?

2. With regard to your multicultural experience, was there more homogeneity (mostly a's and b's) or more diversity (mostly c's, d's, and e's) in your answers? Explain.

3. Was there a difference between your multicultural experiences in your early life (items 1–8) and your present life (items 9–16)? Please explain.

4. How satisfied are you with your level of engagement with diversity?

5. What actions if any would you like to take to improve your level of involvement in multicultural experiences?

WHY IS MULTICULTURAL RESPONSIBILITY IMPORTANT?

Students come to college campuses from a wide range of racial, ethnic, and cultural backgrounds. The mission statements or values of colleges often reflect the idea of multicultural responsibility. Consider the following mission statements from various universities and community colleges in the United States:

- The University ". . . fosters a multicultural environment in which the dignity and rights of the individual are respected. Intellectual diversity, integrity, and disciplined inquiry in the search for knowledge are of paramount importance." (University of Kansas)

- "The college provides open access and innovative learning systems to respond to the ever-changing needs and interests of a diverse and dynamic community." (Howard Community College)

- We foster ". . . cultural, ethnic, racial, and gender diversity in the faculty, staff and student body." (University System of Georgia; Albany State University, Clayton State University, and Gordon College)

- We ". . . value diversity because it enhances our education and because it provides tools to be culturally respectful, professionally competent, and civically responsible. **Respect.** We encourage respect, humanity, and integrity in our treatment of each other, and we care for the well being and safety of others. **Responsibility.** We have a responsibility to society to contribute to its social, cultural, political, aesthetic, ethical, and economic well being. **Truth.** We honor and impart principles of academic honesty, freedom, truth, and integrity." (Oregon State University)

Clearly, the goal of many colleges is to create a diverse population from whom all students can learn from each other and have an enriching multicultural experience. While this goal is noble, it will not be achieved by simply bringing people from different backgrounds and cultures together without some well planned, organized procedures and institutional practices designed to help students become multiculturally responsible. Without intentional planning, placing people from different cultures together can create racial conflict, anger, confusion, marginality, and many negative emotions. This array of emotions arises because, while some people will want to increase cross-cultural dialogue, others will be resistant to this. Further complications come from well-intentioned people, who are nonetheless unaware of how to have appropriate and respectful cross-cultural dialogues. In light of these scenarios, becoming an MRP will serve students well. Some of the benefits of becoming multiculturally responsible follow:

DEFINITION

Marginality is the state of being a marginal person, someone who is not part of the mainstream society or is on the fringe of society. The effects of marginality are often negative and include feelings of shame or rejection from mainstream society.

- You will develop a better understanding of others.
- You will take steps to promote greater harmony among individuals in any setting.
- You will be able to interact with diverse individuals.
- You will be receptive to different cultures, traditions, experiences, beliefs, and ideas.
- You will be able to listen and respond non-judgmentally to others.
- You will have the capacity to avoid generalizing when viewpoints and experiences differ from your own.
- You will be able to function better in an American society that is becoming increasingly diverse and in an increasingly interconnected, global world.

Multicultural Responsibility Index

Being multiculturally responsible means moving beyond talking about multicultural sensitivity to being more accountable for one's actions. At this point, please assess how multiculturally responsible you believe you are by responding to the following statements about yourself.

Multiculturally Responsible Index (MRI)

DIRECTIONS: To the left of each statement indicate your response, where 1 represents *never* and 10 represents *always*.

____10____ I am aware of my own racial/ethnic/cultural identity and how that identity affects my outlook on life.

___8___ I value races/ethnicities/cultures other than my own.

___8___ I have meaningful and ongoing relationships with people from racial/ethnic/cultural groups other than my own.

___8___ I share my resources (skills, time, expertise) with people from racial/ethnic/cultural groups other than my own.

___8___ I am consistently expanding my circle of friends to include individuals from racial, ethnic, and cultural groups other than my own

___5___ I see myself as neither superior nor inferior to other groups.

___10___ I strive to achieve a nonbiased identity.

What is your overall MRI score (70 is the highest possible score)? Which were your highest and lowest item scores? Explain what your scores mean to a selected friend. What are your next steps?

Awareness of your current multicultural responsibility status is an important first step toward becoming a more multiculturally responsible individual. Because we believe that awareness without action is less valuable than action, we strongly encourage you to engage in specific actions toward becoming a more multiculturally responsible individual.

WHY AREN'T WE ALL MULTICULTURALLY RESPONSIBLE?

Many factors and forces hinder students from becoming multiculturally responsible. Some of these hindering forces include: (a) socialization, (b) systemic inequities, (c) prejudice and discrimination, and (d) stereotypical attitudes and biases. These four factors intertwine, making it difficult and more challenging for students to become multiculturally responsible.

Socialization

In the 28 years that I (Max Parker) have taught a course in Multicultural Counseling, White students constantly tell me that they had almost no contact with people from different racial/ethnic/cultural groups until they arrived at college. Some students have reported that their neighborhoods, schools, churches, and the majority of their life experiences have been with members of their own racial/ethnic/cultural groups. It is not uncommon to hear some White students say they have had little or no contact with racial/ethnic/cultural minorities, that they could not describe other groups without using stereotypes, and that they certainly have not had friendships with

---

DEFINITION

Socialization is the process of adapting to the people who inhabit one's surroundings. Socialization continues throughout life, but adaptation to one's own surroundings happens primarily during childhood.

---

students who were from different groups. Understanding one's own socialization is an important first step in becoming multiculturally aware. However, examining one's childhood through a multicultural lens may be threatening and overwhelming for some people. As such, we (Max Parker, an African-American man, and Jennifer Sager, a Jewish-American woman) will share our own socialization experiences to exemplify the importance of personal history in becoming multiculturally responsible.

Like the White students described in the previous paragraph, Max's contact with racial/ethnic/cultural groups outside of his own African-American group was limited, distant, and often negative. In the small rural town where he grew up, he worked in the fields beside Mexican migrant workers but was unable to communicate with them, though he was curious about their language and wished he could speak it. Max had hardly any contact with the Creek Indians in the area, who were isolated on the nearby reservation. All he knew about them was that they worked hard and enjoyed hunting and fishing. White people, on the other hand, Max had been taught to fear. Having grown up in an all Black community, Max never knew a White person of his own age— not even a fellow athlete. To satisfy his curiosity about White football players, he watched their games through a knothole in a wooden fence around the football stadium that Black people were not allowed to enter prior to the Civil Rights Movement of the 1960s and 1970s. He made imaginary friends with two White football players who played the same position he played.

Max's first personal contact with White people occurred when he attended Stillman, a small private college that had a Black student body and a majority of White professors. He recalls feeling paralyzed when in the presence of Whites for the first time. He had been socialized to fear White people, to obey them, and to see them as superior. Such perceptions were clearly impediments to rapport and to building multicultural relations. These negative

---

DEFINITION

African American or *Black*? The terms used for Black individuals have changed dramatically over the past 50 years. In current usage, the term *African American* refers to those American individuals who have an African heritage. Although there are White individuals who have an African heritage, we are using the term *African American* to refer exclusively to individuals who are Black and have an African heritage. The term *Black* is more inclusive, because it includes those individuals with an African heritage as well as those from Caribbean countries such as Haiti and Jamaica and other parts of the world. Because both terms are commonly used in America today, we will use the terms interchangeably throughout this book.

perceptions began to change when he met Margaret Davis, his Spanish-language teacher at Stillman College. Ms. Davis spent hours with him, not only teaching him basic skills in Spanish, but also helping him to believe in himself, in his abilities to be successful, and in his ability to make a contribution to the betterment of society. Having this positive experience coupled with other positive experiences with Whites in a variety of settings has served to balance or to counteract negative experiences from his early life.

Jennifer grew up in Queens, New York, and was surrounded by a complex arrangement of friends. She remembers learning about Catholicism from her Italian friend, Buddhism from her Asian-American friend, and Judaism from her parents. Her parents taught her to appreciate Black culture through jazz, because they felt that it was the only truly American art form. Jennifer learned from her parents that she should not judge people by their skin color, ethnicity, or culture. This encouraged her to try to be "colorblind." However, in trying to remain colorblind, she often ignored race, ethnicity, and culture altogether. It was years before she learned that colorblindness was an underhanded form of prejudice, that she was "white washing" everything in bleach until there was nothing unique to appreciate about diverse individuals. Included in her colorblindness was her own Jewish culture. She eventually learned that seeing color, but not judging it, was an important way to gain respect and appreciation for other people.

As the authors' experiences show, each person has his or her

> ### DEFINITION
>
> *Native American* or *American Indian*? As we know, Christopher Columbus mislabeled the American people "Indians" when he arrived at what he thought was the "Indies." The term *Native American* was later created to avoid confusion between the indigenous people of America and the indigenous people of India, although some people feel more comfortable with the term *American Indian*. Alaskan Native people (such as the Eskimos and Aleuts) are also included in the term *Native American*. More recently, Native Hawaiians and Pacific Islanders have been included under the *Native American* umbrella term. Because it is the most commonly used term in America today, we will use the term *Native American* throughout this book.

> ### DEFINITION
>
> *Asian American* or *Indian American*? Once the term *Oriental* was used to describe Asian people, but that term is now widely regarded as racist (*Asian* is for people, whereas *Oriental* is for rugs). The precise use of the word *Asian* is very complex. The term **Asian American** typically refers to an American person originally from or whose ancestors are from Korea, Japan, China, Indonesia, Vietnam, Cambodia, the Philippines, and other Asian countries. Although India is technically a part of South Asia, Americans of Indian background are generally referred to as **Indian American** (not to be confused with American Indian). Recently, the Internet term *AZN* has gained in popularity with some Asian-American youth. We will use the terms *Asian American* and *Indian American* throughout this book.

REFLECTION

We all have our own socialization process. What is your personal history? If you feel safe, discuss this with your friends, classmates, or coworkers.

own socialization process. Many of the people we heard from via an Internet research survey conducted to help facilitate the writing of this book stated that their early childhood experiences affected their ability to become multiculturally responsible. One of the respondents, Carlos, a Hispanic-American male, wrote:

> I was brought up in a home where African Americans were disliked because of an incident that my mother had with an African-American male. That colored her perceptions of African American people, and of course I incorporated some of those ideas. It took me a long time (years) to overcome these ideas. Exposure and closeness to African Americans helped greatly in changing these ideas.

As with Carlos's story, it is important to remember that socialization is not solely a White/Black issue. Family biases occur in all families. Lori, a 41-year-old European American, poignantly told us how socialization can immobilize people, and pointed out the importance of personal awareness in increasing our multicultural responsibility.

DEFINITION

European American or *White? European American* refers to individuals who link their heritage back to Europe. These people are most often White; however, this term expresses their ethnic heritage, rather than their skin tone. *White* refers to someone's skin tone. Having a White racial identity also includes the privilege that exists with being part of the majority culture in America. Because both terms are commonly used in America today, we will use them interchangeably throughout this book.

Where we come from has some influence on how we see and process information. Perhaps, albeit unintentionally, we had parents who were raised to think narrow-mindedly, or perhaps we had limited opportunity to be integrated with folks "different than ourselves" due to geographic or other social constraints. Without a reason to question, or a critical incident to prompt personal questioning, there might not be a motivation to know about the responsibility to grow in sensitivity.

REFLECTION

As you began to do in the Multicultural Experience Inventory exercise, think about your childhood history a little more deeply. In what ways were you socialized to think negatively about other racial/ethnic/cultural groups?

Our personal history is a key component in becoming multiculturally responsible. The exploration of our childhood socialization helps us to understand ourselves better and helps us to know what changes we need to make toward becoming multiculturally responsible. Mathias and

French (1996) suggest that families need to trace their history of prejudice by spending time recalling how parents and grandparents responded to different races, ethnicities, and cultures. Most important, Mathias and French challenge people to ask how their family's prejudice has influenced their own personal behavior. Otherwise, people may be repeating old habits without being conscious of their prejudices.

Systemic Inequities

Systemic inequities, like socialization, are another life challenge for becoming multiculturally responsible. On most of the predominantly White, public college campuses, some of the following examples of systemic inequity are instantly observable:

- The majority of the students, faculty, and administrators at most colleges are White. For example, during the 2000s, one particular campus had 81 full-time minority faculty out of 2,746 overall full-time faculty (Stewart-Dowdell & McCarthy, 2003).

- In many colleges (particularly in those states where protective civil rights laws do not exist) LGBT student groups have difficulty obtaining funding from the university, whereas hobby-oriented groups such as chess clubs and other groups have no such problems.

- In 2004, only 5% of presidents of Division I-A universities were minorities. About 84% were White males (Lapchick, 2004).

- Although the Americans with Disabilities Act has improved matters substantially, many college campuses continue to hold classes in buildings with limited access for students with disabilities.

- Although a high percentage of the football players are students of color, head coaches are typically White. For example, University of Central Florida's Institute for Diversity and Ethics in Sport reported that as of October 2004, there were five Black individuals and one Latino individual employed as head coaches at the 117 Division I-A football schools (Lapchick, 2004). In fact, prior to 2004, there were no Black coaches in the Southeastern Conference. By comparison, about 43 percent of the football players in Division I-A are Black.

These longstanding inequities are also referred to as systemic inequities. Many people in the Internet survey we conducted wrote

> **DEFINITION**
>
> The term *systemic inequities* refers to racial, ethnic, and cultural inequalities that are caused by system-wide problems rather than by individual prejudices. For instance, under-funding of schools in poor neighborhoods compared with schools in wealthy neighborhoods is an inequality caused by a problematic educational system.

about systemic inequities at their own schools that affect the cultural development of their students.

- Tom, a 33-year-old White professor, said, "Perhaps a better answer is a lack of commitment from the administration for multicultural training activities and increased diversity in the faculty, staff, administration, and student population. If the commitment were there from the very top and it were infused at every level (staff/faculty hiring, student retention, classroom content, funding for multicultural events, etc.) that would help to alleviate a few roadblocks!"

- Jean-Paul, a 32-year-old Mexican-American professor, told us, "There is little commitment by institutions to support individuals for becoming multiculturally responsible unless the institution will make money off of it."

- Elizabeth, a 50-year-old European-American professor, stated, "Our structure for education, and especially higher education, is a top-down, hierarchical, and power-based process. Unless you have some privilege, why would anyone want to subject himself or herself to that unless they are in the dominant group? In addition, our geographic area is very homogenous; it is uncomfortable for many people of color to be here. We are not only very White, but also very Protestant, very conventional, and very limited in exposure to different lifestyles. There is a culture of general mistrust of *Others*, or at least a lack of curiosity, because becoming more different is not socially rewarded."

- Helen, a 54-year-old European-American professor, said, "School systems allow students to ridicule others who are different, particularly those struggling with their own sexual orientation or identity."

- Mary, a 49-year-old Latina professor, clearly stated, "Our world is a White world. *Education is a White world system*. Although attempts are being made, mostly by people of color, to integrate the educational system, it remains a rather linear, goal-directed endeavor. So we educate our students from that base."

While professors are often aware of systemic inequities, students may not think about their college as a system. Despite this lack of awareness, systemic inequities can negatively affect students. Systemic inequities give all people involved with the institution the perception that the majority is the desired population, and that all minorities (racial, ethnic, cultural) are not valued as highly.

Exercise for Examining Systemic Inequities on Your Campus

Nearly all colleges today are doing hard work to combat inequality on campus. But certain systemic inequities may be hard to surmount despite their best efforts. In this exercise you are asked to examine some of the systemic inequities that may exist on your campus. The purpose is to show how deeply cemented systemic inequities can be, even on the most progressive campuses.

Spend some time making some observations about your campus and browsing through your college guidebook/course guide. Keep the following questions in mind:

1. How diverse is the student body of your college? Does the racial, ethnic, and cultural makeup of students at your college closely resemble the diversity of the country as a whole, or are minority groups on campus a smaller minority than they are in America as a whole?

2. How diverse is the faculty at your college? Does the racial, ethnic, cultural, and gender makeup of the faculty accurately reflect the diversity of the country as a whole, or does the faculty tend to be mostly White, mostly European American, and mostly men?

3. How many of the coaches of the various athletic teams at your college are minorities or women? How does this balance with the number of minority players on those teams? Are all of the men's teams coached by men? Are all of the women's teams coached by women?

4. Is a wide variety of courses in African-American studies, gay and lesbian studies, Asian-American studies, Hispanic studies, Native-American studies, etc., offered at your college, or are just a few such diversity-oriented courses offered? Furthermore, if you are on a large campus, can you receive a minor (or a major) in diversity studies or simply a certificate/concentration in a diversity area?

If you find that any of the areas above appear unequal at your college, these problems are probably systemic rather than a result of attempts by the college administration to prevent diversity. Despite efforts to attract minority students, faculty, and both minority and women coaches, system-wide factors such as lack of programs for women coaches in training across the country or shortage of scholarships to attract economically disadvantaged students may prevent true diversity from existing on college campuses today.

What makes this particular roadblock more difficult to handle than problems caused by socialization is that systemic inequities often appear to be too big for people to take on and too difficult to change, so that people feel defeated by the system in striving to become multiculturally responsible. Individuals within the system may feel stifled by imagining that being multiculturally appropriate suffices, but may feel unable to go the extra step to becoming multiculturally responsible. It is true that a system may feel too big to take on, but sometimes taking on a piece of the system will make a difference. For example, instead of asking, "Why are there no disability awareness programs on campus?" begin by asking, "How could there be more disability awareness programs on campus; what would it look like if there were disabilities programs?"

Prejudice and Discrimination

Another hindering force to multicultural responsibility on campus is prejudice and discrimination. Prejudice and discrimination can be blatant or passive. We are all able to easily recognize blatant prejudice and discrimination.

> **DEFINITION**
>
> ***Multiculturally appropriate*** versus ***multiculturally responsible.*** There is a key difference between being multiculturally appropriate and being multiculturally responsible. Being multiculturally responsible means being accountable for something as big or as challenging as systemic inequality, while being multiculturally appropriate means intellectualizing diversity or simply giving "lip service" to the issue without concrete action. In addition, it means being politically correct by saying all the right things about diversity such as "appreciating differences," "people are more alike than they are different," or "I do not see color; everyone should be treated the same," but without the commitment to make systemic changes.

> **REFLECTION**
>
> What are some ways that you could change your campus system? What would you like to see done differently?

> **DEFINITION**
>
> ***Prejudice*** and ***discrimination***. There is a fundamental difference between prejudice and discrimination. A *prejudice* is a "pre-judgment," or a negative attitude toward a particular racial, ethnic, or cultural group that is not based on rational thought. *Discrimination* is an action, in which prejudicial attitudes are put into practice.

As shorthand, these blatant prejudices are sometimes referred to as "isms." A blatantly discriminatory person would make a concerted effort to prevent someone from a particular group from enjoying the same rights as others.

Although blatant prejudice and discrimination do still exist on college campuses and elsewhere, college students do not experience them as often as did people in previous generations. However, individuals should be careful of passive prejudice and discrimination, which can be just as harmful and harder to spot and therefore combat. Passive prejudice is a result of people not being fully aware of their prejudices. Passive discrimination is lack of action based on this lack of awareness. For example, passively prejudicial individuals might believe in the notion that everything is better now than it was in the past, therefore they may be passively discriminatory by neglecting to take action when they witness discriminatory behaviors. In short, passive prejudice and discrimination are forms of complacency, which is a major threat to the advancement of diverse relations. Passive prejudice and discrimination can come in the form of shutting down conversation by being oblivious to the inequity between people or by limiting conversation by simply ignoring difference. Instead of avoiding difference there should be an attempt to make people's differences the primary lens through which they are seen and respected. Following are some examples of passive prejudice and passive discrimination.

> **DEFINITION**
>
> ***Isms*** is shorthand for describing several forms of prejudice such as racism, sexism, and heterosexism. Other forms of isms can include bias against older people (ageism) or people with disabilities (ableism). Not all isms contain the same "-ism" suffix. For example, other forms of isms include misogyny (hatred of women), homophobia (fear or hatred of gays, lesbians, and bisexuals), and transphobia (fear or hatred of transgender individuals).

1. Passive prejudice: Assuming that race relations in the United States have improved to the point that everybody has the same opportunities.

Passive discrimination: Working against affirmative action, because if all people regardless of race, ethnicity, and culture now have the same opportunities, minorities should not be provided with unfair advantages.

2. Passive prejudice: Believing that lesbian, gay, bisexual, and transgender rights have advanced enough so that there is no reason for the LGBT community to be asking for more.

Passive discrimination: Refusing to listen to arguments about legalizing gay marriage or making the adoption of children by same-sex couples more feasible because those are "special rights," not basic rights.

3. Passive prejudice: Believing that men and women are now on a completely equal playing field in the workplace.

Passive discrimination: Arguing that women who complain of sexual harassment or job discrimination in the workplace today are unfairly trying to get ahead by causing trouble.

Passive prejudices and discriminatory behaviors are hard to combat, because holding people accountable for not taking action seems backwards. The best we can do as MRPs in training is to recognize and argue against the types of arguments that lead to passive discrimination whenever we encounter them.

Exercise for Recognizing Your Own Passive Prejudices

DIRECTIONS: Answer the following questions using a scale of 1 to 5, with 1 meaning "completely disagree," 2 meaning "disagree somewhat," 3 meaning "neither agree nor disagree," 4 meaning "agree somewhat," and 5 meaning "completely agree."

1. Aside from occasional sexist comments, women no longer have to deal with discrimination in the workplace, and the long-existing wage discrepancy between men and women workers performing the same jobs is now a thing of the past.

2. Lesbian, gay, bisexual, and transgender people now have equal rights in all states, except for marriage rights, for which they are now fighting.

3. The stereotype of the service professions being made up mostly of minority workers is now a thing of the past. The proportion of minorities to whites in the service professions is now about the same as the proportion of minorities to whites in the population as a whole.

4. All workplaces in the country are now fully accessible to disabled persons, so there is no reason for disabled people to encounter difficulties being accommodated in the modern workplace.

If you answered mostly 4s or 5s to the statements above, you have some research to do in order to combat passive prejudices you hold to be true. The fact is that none of the above statements are true: women still do not earn as much as men and often experience workplace discrimination, particularly in certain professions that remain male dominated. Lesbian, gay, and bisexual people have equal workplace rights in only a few states and cities across the United States, and in some states can be fired for no reason. Transgender individuals rarely have equal workplace rights. The low-paying service professions are still very disproportionately held by minority workers. Despite the Americans with Disabilities Act, many workspaces are still not up to the standards to accommodate workers with disabilities.

Stereotyping

The last factor hindering multicultural responsibility is stereotyping. Stereotypes are often learned during childhood, and they allow us to support our prejudices. For instance, if people believe the stereotype that individuals from Colombia tend to be drug dealers, then they will remember news stories involving Colombian individuals as drug dealers, but forget news stories that involve White individuals as drug dealers or Colombian individuals who are business people, educators, or entertainers. The stereotype feeds the prejudice and continues in a self-repeating fashion.

> ### DEFINITION
>
> *Stereotyping* is making simplistic, generalized assumptions about people in other racial/ethnic/cultural groups because that is less challenging and more convenient than appreciating people as complex human beings.

People in our Internet study wrote about stereotyping and bias and how it affects them in their daily lives:

- *Estaban*, a biracial college student, stated, "Stereotyping might make people unable to mingle with other cultures because they are afraid of changes or differences. I think someone should embrace those rather than run away from the differences."

- Romena, a Hispanic-American graduate student, said, "People tend to deny any biases they have, and when they are aware of social injustice, they think someone else should do something about it."

To help you become more aware of your own stereotypes, one useful route to take is to pinpoint exactly what those stereotypes are. Once you identify the stereotypes that you hold true, you will realize how much you take them to heart, and you can then work to eliminate them.

> **REFLECTION**
>
> Can you recall an experience when you were clearly guilty of stereotyping? What were the consequences of it? What can you do to reduce your frequency of stereotyping?

Exercise for Recognizing Stereotypes

DIRECTIONS: Complete the following exercise as quickly as possible. Try not to think critically about or rationalize your answers. A bias is often an automatic thought. For each of the following phrases, list as many groups (racial, ethnic, cultural, and gender) as you think fit into each category or are stereotypically believed to fit into each category.

blonde	unintelligent/low IQ
Asian	intellectual
_A.A._	lazy/bad work ethic
Asian	driven/motivated
Asian	cheap/frugal
White	generous/giving
White	good lovers/sexy
_A.A._	bad lovers/un-sexy
	sexually repressed
	sexually promiscuous
	uptight/stiff
	casual/laid back
_A.A._	criminal/dangerous
	upstanding/trustworthy

_____Asian_____	bad grasp of English
_____	articulate/well-spoken
_____	musically inclined/artistic
_____	unclean/poor hygiene
_____	clean/immaculate
_____	convenience store owner
_____	service worker
_____	janitor/cleaning crew worker
_____	computer whiz/scientist
_____women_____	homemaker
_____	interior designer
_____	lawyer
_____Jewish_____	doctor
_____white_____	president of company
_____	good dancer/rhythmic
_____asian_____	can't dance/no sense of rhythm
_____	nurturing
_____	aggressive/pushy
_____	complaining/whiny
_____	wealthy/upper class
_____	poor/lower class
_____	humorous/funny
_____	lacking humor/overly serious
_____	bad at sports/uncoordinated
_____	good at sports/athletic
_____	fashion conscious
_____	fashion challenged
_____	politically correct
_____	politically dangerous/terrorist

At this point, do not share your answers. Simply take some time and think about these stereotypes. Where did you learn these things? Did someone teach you these values? Could you have misinterpreted events in your life to support these statements? Do you agree with these statements?

Even those who are trained to value other races, ethnicities, and cultures may sometimes fall victim to their own stereotypes, despite good intentions. Throughout this book, your stereotypes will be challenged. Real change can occur only if you are willing to let go of your stereotypes and replace them with the idea that other groups are as valuable and diverse as your own.

> **QUOTATION**
>
> *The greatest discovery of my generation is that human beings can alter their lives by altering their attitudes of mind.*
>
> WILLIAM JAMES

Negative stereotyping or labeling is detrimental because it hinders human development in general and in particular is a threat to the achievement of human potential. People rarely engage in this behavior on purpose. However, in our society, individuals constantly make judgments about others either consciously or unconsciously whenever people interact. We believe that the most devastating effect of stereotyping occurs when individuals buy into or internalize the stereotypes. For example, the stereotype that women cannot do mathematics is fairly harmless until women begin to believe that they cannot do math. The stereotype that Black and Hispanic-American students cannot excel

> **REFLECTION**
>
> How do you stereotype yourself? Are there ways that you are limiting yourself in regards to academic or social choices? What would you do if you were not afraid of failure?

academically in college has less power than it does if these students buy into the notion that they cannot learn as well as their White counterparts.

Unfortunately, many people are stressed and depressed because they have internalized the stereotypes that pervade every aspect of the American society. If this is true, it is incumbent upon multiculturally responsible students, faculty, and administrators to create campus environments that are culturally sensitive, to counteract the powerful dynamics of the myriad stereotypes that exist.

AWARENESS INTO ACTION: TAKING THE TIME AND MAKING THE EFFORT TO BECOME MULTICULTURALLY RESPONSIBLE

Jennifer, one of the authors, witnessed an incident that involved an elderly Black woman asking someone to repeat what a speaker said about genetics. The White woman to her right began to give her the definition of the word *genetics*. The Black woman responded sharply with, "I know the meaning of the word—I did not hear what she said!" Clearly, the Black woman felt talked down to and the White woman was unaware of her patronizing behavior. Ironically, this incident happened on a planning committee for a race relations conference, and these two people had been members for years!

This example demonstrates that even though some people are willing to make the effort to be involved in multiculturally responsible activities, they need to continue to do personal work and take time out of their busy schedules to make an impact. Following are a few quotations from our Internet survey that speak to the importance of putting time and effort into becoming an MRP.

- Jim, a 57-year-old African American, felt that "One of the limiting factors is a tendency for people not to reach out to understand or learn about others. For the most part, we all have our agendas, work schedules, and classes to attend. There is no immediate need or impetus to stretch out and make new acquaintances or learn about others. For students, offering a curriculum of courses that expose them to multicultural issues might be a benefit."

- Carol, a 27-year-old therapist, stated, "When a person stays within his or her own cultural group, opportunity may not arise to become multiculturally responsible."

- Melissa, a 30-year-old psychologist, wrote: "I see fear as being the #1 block to multicultural responsibility—fear of being exposed for one's beliefs and being rejected because of them, and fear of losing power to those who are different from oneself. Other road blocks are lack of opportunity or initiative to have exposure to those who are different from oneself and lack of energy/burnout regarding these issues."

Yes, everyone is busy. Yes, people are afraid of the unknown. Change has always taken time and strength. There are many roadblocks to becoming multiculturally responsible: childhood socialization, systemic inequality, prejudice and discrimination, and stereotypes. It is important to understand that becoming multiculturally responsible is a time-consuming and sometimes challenging process, but well worth it.

CHAPTER AND PERSONAL REVIEW QUESTIONS

1. What is the difference between race, ethnicity, and culture? How do these terms interweave with each other?

2. Why is the pursuit of multicultural responsibility an important endeavor?

3. Having completed a variety of exercises related to multicultural responsibility and learned about a variety of topics related to the subject, rate on a scale of 1 to 10 (with 1 being the least multiculturally responsible and 10 being the most multiculturally responsible) where you feel you currently fall on the scale. Do you feel confident that you can do better?

4. What are the four major roadblocks to multicultural responsibility covered in this chapter?

5. What are the preferred terms used to describe the various racial, ethnic, and cultural groups discussed in this chapter? Why are those the preferred terms?

6. In what ways does socialization affect multicultural awareness and responsibility?

7. In what ways do systemic inequalities affect multicultural awareness and responsibility?

8. What is the difference between multicultural appropriateness and multicultural responsibility? Why is the distinction of the two terms important?

9. What is the difference among the terms *prejudice, discrimination,* and *stereotyping*? In what ways do each of these factors inhibit multicultural responsibility?

10. List and define as many "isms" as you can. Are there any other "isms" you are aware of that weren't defined in the chapter?

11. Having read this chapter and explored your multicultural awareness somewhat, are you motivated to become an MRP? Explain.

REFERENCES

Lapchick, R. (2004). *Lack of diversity among campus, conference leaders at Division IA schools may contribute to lack of diversity in head football coaching positions*. Research study from the Institute of Diversity and Ethics in Sports and the University of Central Florida. Retrieved February 8, 2005, from http://www.bus.ucf.edu/sport/public/ides/media.htx.

Mathias, B., & French, M. A. (1996). *Forty ways to raise a nonracist child*. New York, NY: HarperCollins Publishers.

Parker, W., Archer J., & Scott, J. (1992). *Multicultural relations on campus: A personal growth approach*. Philadelphia, PA: Accelerated Development.

Ramirez, M. (1991). *Psychotherapy and counseling with minorities: A cognitive approach to individual and cultural differences.* New York, NY: Pergamon Press.

Stewart-Dowdell, B. J., & McCarthy, K. M. (2003). *African Americans at the University of Florida: The past, the present, the future.* University of Florida publication.

CHAPTER 2

Understanding Your Racial, Ethnic, and Cultural Identity

BEFORE YOU READ

1. What do you think the term *racial identity* means (and consequently *ethnic identity* and *cultural identity*?) What do you think the differences might be among these various types of identity?

2. Do White, heterosexual, Protestant males have racial, ethnic, and/or cultural identities? Why or why not?

3. In Chapter 1 we defined the terminology preferred by people from various racial and ethnic groups (Native Americans, African Americans/Blacks, European Americans/Whites, Asian Americans, Latino(a)/ Hispanic Americans, etc.) and those terms that should not be used to describe them. In this chapter we will define the terminology preferred by people from three cultural groups. What do you think are the descriptive terms preferred by people who are attracted to members of their own gender (or both genders); people who feel that they are between or across genders; and people who use wheelchairs, are blind, have attention deficit disorder, or are otherwise different from the majority in terms of physical or mental traits?

INTRODUCTION

Step one to becoming a multiculturally responsible participant (MRP), as discussed in Chapter 1, is to figure out where we each fit within the multicultural puzzle. We have already explored why multicultural responsibility is important, outlined the principal roadblocks that get in the way of multicultural responsibility on campus (socialization, systemic inequality, prejudice and discrimination, and stereotyping), and defined some of the various racial, ethnic, and cultural groups that exist in our society. As you have seen and will see further in subsequent chapters, everyone is part of a racial, ethnic, and/or cultural group (and yes, that includes White, Protestant, Anglo-Saxon, heterosexual males), so we all have our own identities to explore on the way to coexisting with people from racial, ethnic, and cultural identities different from our own. Developing our own identities will be the focus of this chapter. First, we'll discuss racial identity as set forth in the Helms' Racial Identity Development Model. Then, we'll apply the model to non-racial groups, specifically to ethnic and cultural groups. Finally, we'll provide some action plans to facilitate moving from early to more fully realized stages in the identity development process.

RACIAL IDENTITY DEVELOPMENT

There are only a few words in the English language that conjure up more fear, anxiety, and apprehension than the word *race*. Some children grow up hearing parents say, "We do not talk about race in this family." If there is one idea that Americans have consciously or unconsciously attempted to "sweep under the rug," it is the issue of racial differences. Since the Civil War in the United States, there appears to be a collective minimization of the importance of race. The Williams sisters, who are Black Americans and are among the top women tennis players in the world, are often not applauded by White Americans even when the sisters' opponents are from other countries. Yet it is argued that the Williams sisters are disliked not because of their race but rather, because their father, who is their coach, is perceived by some as arrogant. Why does White America not applaud the success of two of its country's biggest champions?

In diversity training workshops, participants are often asked a variety of questions concerning their goals, interests, and personal development toward becoming multiculturally sensitive and skilled. The one question with which many have the greatest difficulty and the question that seems to stun or paralyze them is "What is your racial identity and what does it mean to be a member of your racial group?" White individuals most often say that they are German, Irish, Italian, or some other nationality, but rarely do they identify themselves as White. For some reason these participants are hesitant to discuss issues of race in general and to identify themselves as White in particular. However, this hesitancy to discuss race will change as people explore and progress in their racial identity development.

Janet Helms (1992), a social scientist and a close observer of race relations, believes that the race problem in this country has not been solved and that many White people are not aware of the impact of race or may even deny that racism exists. In her book, *Race Is a Nice Thing to Have*, she wrote:

> Whites seem to be the only racial group that spends more time and effort wondering about the implications of race for other groups than it does for itself. White people have difficulty accepting that they have a race and therefore are threatened by groups who have no such difficulty. Likewise, they seem to have no models for thinking about Whiteness as a healthy part of themselves.

What Is Racial Identity?

It has been our experience and our belief that racial identity is a genuinely dynamic force in the lives of college students that influences their college selection, the friends with whom they choose to associate, their group identity, activities in which they decide to participate, and their general sense of well-being. To illustrate the dynamics of racial identity, consider the true story (names and details have been changed to protect identity) in the following section.

Hong's Experience and Andrew's Experience

Hong Yong-Min, an Asian-American high school senior, was among the top five of the brightest graduates of his class, despite having been born in Korea and having had to overcome a language barrier when he first moved to the United States at age 10. With excellent leadership skills and as one of the most popular students in his school, Hong was elected president of his senior class in a school that was predominantly White.

Even though Hong was a member of a racial

DEFINITION

Racial identity is a term that can be defined in a number of ways. As such, we present a multipart definition:

- The manner or the extent to which one identifies with her or his racial group (Helms, 1995).
- A reflection of how close to or how far from one's racial group a person feels.
- An intuitive or a subjective judgment about the degree that one accepts or rejects her or his racial group.
- A description of how Asian-American, African-American, Hispanic-American, Native-American, or European-American individuals perceive themselves to be.
- An estimation of how important race is to an individual.
- Part of the self-concept related to membership within a racial group.

A dynamic and ever changing force in one's life that is influenced by many factors (Helms, 1995).

minority group, no mention was ever made of his racial minority status as an Asian American. He never talked about the fact that he was Asian American, nor did his mostly White friends. Hong was raised in an upper-middle-class White neighborhood where his father was a medical doctor and his mother owned an antique import business. Most of his family's friends were White. Only English was spoken in the home except when there were visits from his grandmother. One thing that displeased his grandmother was that her grandson never spoke Korean anymore. After years of complaining, she finally conceded that her grandson was becoming so Americanized that he could never be a true transmitter of Korean culture.

Upon graduation from high school, Hong was admitted to his state's predominantly White college where he was expected to become a medical doctor as his father had. To his surprise, Hong was assigned a third-year transfer student, a Korean-American roommate, Andrew Lee, whose views and outlook seemed quite different from his. For example, Andrew was raised in a large Korean community where Korean was spoken by 95% of the people. In their room, Andrew switched from speaking English to speaking Korean quite naturally. While Hong understood Korean, he refused to speak it, believing that all Americans should speak English. Andrew's parents called him every day to be sure that he had sufficient food to eat and to be certain that he was safe. Hong thought to himself that Andrew's parents were being overprotective, not allowing their son to separate or individuate from family ties and grow to be an independent self-actualizing individual.

Other differences between these two Korean-American roommates were their religious and social interests. Andrew attended Catholic Mass three or four times per week while Hong rarely attended. "Why do you attend Mass so frequently?" asked Hong, "You go to Mass as often as you attend class."

"Well," replied Andrew, "my family expects me to attend Mass, and besides, I feel almost ashamed and guilty when I do not attend."

"How are your parents going to know whether or not you attend Mass when they are back home and you are here in college?" Hong asked.

"They will know because I am going to tell them. I talk with my parents every day and I tell them everything that I do. That's just what real Koreans do," said Andrew.

Having been introduced to politics in high school, it was natural for Hong to continue his political ambition at the college level. He had heard that one way to become a successful college politician was to gain experience as an officer in student government and improve connections by joining a fraternity. Toward the end of his freshman year Hong prepared himself to join one of the most prestigious White fraternities on campus. First, he changed his name from Hong to John, convincing his roommate and friends to call him by the new Anglicized version of his Korean name. Second, he worked hard to get rid of his still-present accent, with the goal of speaking Midwestern Standard English.

Hong had for a few years after his family's emigration to America continued to speak Korean with his grandmother, who insisted that her only grandson be proud of his Korean culture. However, Hong (John) soon rejected his grand-mother's teachings, believing that holding on to Korean culture was like hold-ing on to relics of the past that have no place in our technological society. "John" joined a White fraternity, was elected to several offices in student gov-ernment, and eventually became the first Asian-American president of the stu-dent body in that college. Hong was unsure if he should invite his family to celebrate this important event in his life, because he knew his grandmother would be disappointed when he spoke only English in his acceptance speech. Hong did not want to be perceived as Korean, feeling that he had assimilated into the majority culture. He felt that speaking Korean would sabotage his achievements. He told others that he wanted his family to be a part of his life, but respect the choices that he had made for himself.

Andrew, on the other hand, maintained close contact with his family and enjoyed regular weekend visits from them. He managed to work through jokes from friends about the huge entourage of grandparents, aunts, uncles, brothers, sisters, nieces, nephews, and parents who made their monthly pil-grimage to campus to visit the son of whom they were very proud. Andrew loved his family and could hardly wait for their frequent visits.

It had been difficult for Andrew to leave home due to the closeness of his family. Rather than attend a four-year university initially, he had decided to attend a community college at home. During his time at the community college, he had excelled and had gained confidence in himself and his aca-demic skills. Although there were ample opportunities to learn about other cultures, Andrew chose to spend the majority of his time learning about his own culture. When he came to the University during his junior year, he sought out other Korean-American students with views similar to his. He joined the Asian-American student organization to provide support for and promote the issues and needs of Asian students on campus. Andrew found a great deal of meaning in his association with the Asian-American or-ganization, eventually seeing them as his family away from home. As the semester progressed, Andrew became curious about other cultures. He at-tended a wheelchair basketball game, a disability awareness event, and a Native-American dance celebration. Andrew began to recognize his limited knowledge about different cultures and struggled with how to balance a connection to his own culture and other cultures.

The Racial Identity Model

We can see through the college experiences of those two Korean-American men that major worldview differences exist within members of the same racial group. The racial identity attitudes of both Hong/John and Andrew parallel the statuses described by **Helms's Racial Identity Development**

DEFINITION

Helms's Racial Identity Development Model:
Five Statuses that People of Color May Express

Pre-Encounter (Conformity): Use of a White American frame of reference to view and think of the world
- Attitudes toward own racial group: Devaluation or nonsalience
- Attitudes toward Whiteness: Idealization, identification, or nonsalience

Encounter (Dissonance): Abandonment of White American frame of reference due to social or personal encounters
- Attitudes toward own racial group: Ambivalence and/or confusion
- Attitudes toward Whiteness: Ambivalence, confusion, and/or criticalness

Immersion/Emersion: Idolization of own "racial groupness" (e.g., Blackness, Asian-ness, etc.), although the extent of true internalization of positive attitudes concerning one's racial group membership can be minimal
- Attitudes toward own racial group: Idealization
- Attitudes toward Whiteness: Denigration and/or rejection

Internalization: Self-acceptance, confidence in individually defined identity, capacity to assess and respond to members of the dominant group
- Attitudes toward own racial group: Acceptance, identification
- Attitudes toward Whiteness: Acknowledgment and/or tolerance

Integrative Awareness: Valuation of one's own collective identity while empathizing and collaborating with members of other oppressed groups

Source: Adapted from Helms, J. E. (1995). An update of Helms' White and people of color racial identity models. In J. G. Ponterotto, J. M. Casas, L. A. Suzuki, & C. M. Alexander (Eds.), *Handbook of multicultural counseling* (pp. 93–122). Thousand Oaks, CA: Sage Publications.

Model. First, Hong's attitudes are similar to the **Pre-encounter** or **Conformity** stage (often characterized by the denial system). Although these statuses are dynamic and ever changing, it is clear that Hong denounces his own culture, prefers White values, and sees the White culture as supreme.

On the other hand, Andrew's attitudes and behaviors are more similar to Stage 3, **Immersion/ Emersion** and Stage 4, **Internalization.** During conversations with Hong, Andrew asserts his own culture and hints that he resists other cultures ("that's what real Koreans do"). However, he becomes interested in other cultural groups, which represents a move toward the Internalization

REFLECTION

In what ways do the experiences of these two Asian-American men help you understand the concept of racial identity? How did their experiences help you to understand your own racial identity?

stage. Individuals in this status have a strong identification with their own racial group and are beginning to recognize some of their biases. Ideally, both Hong and Andrew will move toward the **Integrative Awareness** stage, which focuses on collaboration with members of other oppressed groups, a selective appreciation for the dominant culture, and a developing sense of security and inner peace regarding their racial identity.

Racial Minority Identity Status Exercise

DIRECTIONS: Please examine the following series of questions. Students who identify themselves as members of racial minority groups are asked to respond honestly to each question by circling the number that most closely corresponds to their opinion. 1 means "strongly agree," 2 means "agree," 3 means "neutral," 4 means "disagree," and 5 means "strongly disagree." Students who do not identify themselves as racial minorities are asked to read through the questions in preparation for a group discussion.

1 2 3 4 5   1. Most of my friends are White. I only have a few acquaintances from racial minority groups like myself.

1 2 3 4 5   2. Sometimes I think that the White people with whom I am friends are not always supportive of my being a member of a racial minority group, but I don't know many people from my own race either.

1 2 3 4 5   3. I am sick and tired of White racists. I would prefer to spend time with people from my own race.

1 2 3 4 5   4. I'm moving away from anger toward the oppressors. It just isn't getting anyone anywhere.

1 2 3 4 5   5. I consider myself an activist, working with members of all of the diverse groups in my community to do away with racism and oppression.

1 2 3 4 5   6. The reason White people are successful in life is because they know how to work the system to their advantage better than others.

1 2 3 4 5   7. I feel like a fish out of water. I can't say that I'm happy about either my own mostly minority community or the prospect of moving into a mostly White neighborhood.

1 2 3 4 5   8. I've never wasted my time hanging out with White people and I'm not about to start now.

1 2 3 4 5   9. My White friends are very politically aware, so we manage to have productive conversations about race, even if they sometimes don't get my point of view.

1 2 3 4 5   10. I would be completely comfortable dating and committing long-term to a White person.

1 2 3 4 5   11. My people need to stop whining and move beyond how they are oppressed, because that's the American way.

1 2 3 4 5   12. I think people pretty much determine their own fate, with a little help from outside.

1 2 3 4 5   13. White people listen to the most rigid music. I mean, classical music, heavy metal, soft rock, and punk versus music that comes from the soul and from the community? There's no comparison.

1 2 3 4 5   14. I didn't used to have any White friends, but I've made some good White friends in college with whom I actually have a great deal in common.

1 2 3 4 5   15. I'd prefer to live in a diverse community, where everyone just gets along.

1 2 3 4 5   16. I'm embarrassed that minorities are using the system by collecting welfare and unemployment checks.

1 2 3 4 5   17. White people have caused a lot of problems for minorities, but now they have to deal with reverse discrimination and affirmative action, so I guess it evens out.

1 2 3 4 5   18. White people may read books by Sandra Cisneros, go to Spike Lee movies, and eat at soul food restaurants, but I think it's just lip service to prove they're not racist.

1 2 3 4 5   19. I'm very confident about my racial identity now and can confront racism firmly but without exploding in anger every time.

1 2 3 4 5   20. I am interested in either pursuing a career related to eliminating oppression and social problems, or if I end up doing something else, I definitely plan to give back to the community by volunteering or contributing in some other way.

1 2 3 4 5   21. Race isn't an issue with me. I prefer to just be viewed as a human being.

1 2 3 4 5   22. I'd like to start hanging out with more people from my own race, but I don't have the same interests as most people of my race.

1 2 3 4 5   23. I'm always surprised at how varied people of my race are.

1 2 3 4 5   24. People of my race are just as varied in their interests and outlooks as people from other races. It takes all kinds.

1 2 3 4 5   25. Every person has a stake in making the world a better place for everyone.

The following chart indicates which questions from the preceding list fit with each racial identity status. Those students who have identified themselves as members of racial minorities and completed the questionnaire are asked to put a check mark in the spaces in the chart next to each question to which they responded with a 1 (strongly agree) or 2 (agree). Although this exercise is not scientifically perfect, it should give those students who completed the questionnaire an indication as to where they fit on the racial identity status model. The statuses under which they have put the most check marks indicate approximately where they fall in terms of racial identity status. Once the exercise has been completed, all students are requested to discuss the exercise. Revealing their racial identity status is the students' choice.

Pre-encounter		Encounter		Immersion/ Emersion		Internalization		Integrative Awareness	
1		2		3		4		5	
6		7		8		9		10	
11		12		13		14		15	
16		17		18		19		20	
21		22		23		24		25	

Advancement Toward Integrative Awareness

How does one achieve the Integrative Awareness stage, the most optimal stage of the racial/identity model? A detailed response to this question is beyond the scope of this book and would occupy too much space. However, Helms and Cook (1999) have proposed the following factors as key influences of racial identity:

a. Individual experiences

b. Meaningful events in one's environments

c. Societal and familial messages and images

d. Observations of how group members are treated in society

To highlight important aspects of reaching the Integrative Awareness stage, one of this book's authors, Max, will highlight factors he believes influenced his racial identity status. Like many college students, Max recalls his college years (1959–1963) as a time of self-examination and personal growth in general, and advancements in his racial identity attitudes and behavior in particular. He attended college during the civil rights movement of the late 1950s and early 1960s when protest, revolutionary thought, and activism were common occurrences. In the midst of this, Max began to question his previously held beliefs about himself as a Black male living in a White Southern racist society. He asked himself, "If Rosa Parks, an elderly Black woman, had the courage to sit in the front of the bus, why shouldn't I?" The responsibility to get involved rather than to passively exist dominated his thoughts and disturbed his comfort. Voices of many Black leaders, both historical and contemporary, made him feel uncomfortable in his endorsement of a racial identity status characterized by idealizing White values and denigrating Black values, seeing Whites as superior and seeing himself as inferior, and conforming to the ways of the dominant culture.

REFLECTION

Identify at least one historical figure and one contemporary figure that best represent your cultural group. In which racial identity status are they?

One such leader was Dr. Martin Luther King, Jr., who said, "Stand up against racism wherever it is found." Reverend Jesse Jackson declared, "I am somebody," and Mary McLeod Bethune proclaimed, "My name is Mary McLeod Bethune, I am Negro, I am Black, and I am going somewhere." These voices and others challenged his willingness to accept societal conditions as they were, and encouraged him instead to begin to think of life as it could be.

Throughout his life, Max has been exposed to Black literature, which has served as a dynamic force driving him from seeing himself as being inferior to seeing himself as a person of worth and dignity. Woodson (1933) said, "You have been mis-educated unless you know something about your history." In a message to his nephew Baldwin (1995) wrote, "Know whence you came. If you know whence you came, there is really no limit to where you can go." DuBois (1940) offered wisdom about how to live in the Black world and the White world in America. He said, "It is a peculiar sensation, this double consciousness. One ever feels his two-ness—An American, A Negro; two souls, two thoughts, two irreconcilable strivings, two warring ideals in one dark body, whole dogged strength alone keeps it from being torn asunder."

Max learned from DuBois that he must be able to speak two languages and must be able to crisscross to avoid being stressed out and to avoid being in a constant state of racial conflict. The message that he received from Frederick Douglass was simple but most profound. Mr. Douglass believed that success comes with a struggle and with hard work. African Americans will not receive respect without a major commitment to change and a willingness to stay the course under adverse conditions.

While historical and contemporary role models presented in the literature have enhanced the advancements of his racial identity, Max believes his most profound influence has resulted from personal contact and interactions with a variety of friends across racial and cultural lines. Through personal contact, he has been able to observe firsthand how much other groups have in common with his group. These common qualities among groups have provided Max with myriad opportunities for interpersonal communication, knowledge

---

DEFINITION

Helms's Racial Identity Development Model: Six Statuses That White People May Express

Contact: Unaware about racism
- Learned racial stereotypes may be unintentionally applied
- Cultural standards that favor Whiteness (e.g., beauty, music, art)

Disintegration: Increased awareness of inequality
- Getting in touch with racism, and coping with the lack of support for doing so
- Reactions including shock, avoidance, confusion, helplessness, guilt, and fear

Reintegration: Fearing or resenting people of color; defending White privileges as earned; acting on misinformation, distortions, etc.

Pseudo-Independence: Belief in fairness and Whites' responsibility for ending racism, but distancing oneself through:
- Detaching intellectually from the negative effects of racism
- Focusing on the problems with others rather than the self

Immersion/Emersion: Focusing on one's own role, responsibility, accountability
- Shifting focus from others to the self with emotional engagement
- Moving out of one's comfort zone to understand racism and difference

Autonomy: Lifelong process of defining oneself positively as a White person
- Attempting to interact with the world from a nonracist perspective
- Working to relinquish unearned privileges of racism

Source: Adapted from Helms, J. E. (1995). An update of Helms' White and people of color racial identity models. In J. G. Ponterotto, J. M. Casas, L. A. Suzuki, & C. M. Alexander (Eds.), Handbook of multicultural counseling (pp. 93–122). Thousand Oaks, CA: Sage Publications.

---

acquisition, and anxiety reduction. All of these experiences have interacted to help him advance toward higher levels of racial identity.

White Racial Identity

While earlier models of racial identity focused on people of color, it has been determined that White people also must become aware of their racial identity status. White individuals have their own six statuses, based on Helms's model.

We characterize the first two stages, **Contact** and **Disintegration,** as novice stages. White individuals in these stages are satisfied with the status quo and are oblivious to the existence of other racial groups. When an event such as a class discussion or reading a book on multicultural relations occurs, the individual may deny any internal anxiety. It is during these two stages that a person may say or think, "I am not White." By this, the individuals imply that they do not benefit from being White, defend against

any negative implications that come with being White, and distance themselves from overtly racist people such as those who would belong to racist
organizations. Paul Kivel (2002) explains that people are quick to add another cultural piece, implying that they are not White in order to claim a victim status and avoid responsibility for the current hotbed of American racism.
Yes, it is true that some groups (i.e., Jews, Irish Catholic, Italian) were once
considered not White, but are now considered White. On the West Coast in
1848, Mexicans were considered White, while Chinese were given the same
status as Blacks (Kivel, 2002). Being White is a "constantly shifting boundary
separating those who are entitled to have certain privileges from those whose
exploitation and vulnerability to violence is justified by their not being white"
(Kivel, 2002, p. 15). It is generally true in American society that a person
benefits by having white skin whether she or he is gay, poor, or has disabilities. An individual with a complex culture may have several identities through
which they need to advance, such as White racial identity as well as ethnic
and/or cultural identity (such as sexual orientation identity).

The next two stages of White racial identity, **Reintegration** and **Pseudo-
independence** can be thought of as intermediate stages. In these stages,
the individual idealizes White groups (by this we mean predominantly White
organizations, not racist or White supremacist organizations) and often
judges other racial groups. Pseudo-independence is common among individuals with some higher education, who are knowledgeable of racial issues
and "help" other racial groups, yet when they are made aware of their racial
inappropriateness, their defending responses are often "I have lots of Black
friends" or "I'm very aware of the issues facing minorities in this country."
Individuals in these stages are not considered to be multiculturally responsible. They also tend to engage in lip service and sometimes do not challenge
themselves to reach the final two stages.

The final two stages, **Immersion/Emersion** and **Autonomy,** can be
viewed as advanced stages that reflect multicultural responsibility. These
stages require hard work and a great deal of introspection. People who have
reached these stages have come to a personal understanding of racism and
how they have knowingly or unconsciously contributed to it. These stages
are characterized by the awareness that being White has certain advantages
in our society and by attempts to actively shun these advantages.

Here is an example of how to give up privilege: When one of this book's
authors, Jennifer, is in a store, she is often waited on before people of color,
even though they are physically in front of her! Rather than assuming that
this is her lucky day, she recognizes that she is being helped first because
of her Whiteness and resists this privilege by asking the "invisible" person
if he or she is already waiting. This often creates a conversation with the
"invisible" person and sometimes an alliance. If the salesperson still resists
helping the person of color first, a manager should be called. Do not be
overzealous in enlisting a manager's help, because sometimes your good

intentions can backfire. For instance, Jennifer once called a manager right away when a clerk seemed to be ignoring a Latino customer in front of her. However, it turned out that the "customer" was in fact a friend of the clerk, and so was not waiting in line.

It should be noted that the Helms stages are not set in stone. One has to continue to work on multicultural awareness and action to remain a part of the final two stages. In addition, a critical incident (e.g., car accident with an Asian male, friend going through a bad breakup with a Biracial female) could cause a temporary return to earlier stages. For instance, the 2006 Academy Award winner for best picture, *Crash*, owed its complexity to the fact that characters rapidly shifted between racial identity stages, based on their different racial groups and critical incidents that happened in the film. Only hard work and a firm commitment to multicultural responsibility keep people in the Autonomy stage. The following exercise will help White students identify where they fall on the Helms scale.

White Racial Identity Status Exercise

DIRECTIONS: Please examine the following series of questions. Students who identify themselves as White are asked to respond honestly to each question by circling the number that most closely corresponds to their opinion. 1 means "strongly agree," 2 means "agree," 3 means "neutral," 4 means "disagree," and 5 means "strongly disagree." Students who identify themselves as racial minorities are requested to read through the questions in preparation for a group discussion.

1 2 3 4 5   1. I have had little or no contact with people from racial minority groups in my life.

1 2 3 4 5   2. I'm trying to be more aware of racism, but no one seems to want to give me any credit for trying.

1 2 3 4 5   3. Racial minorities should not be allowed to get into schools unless their grades and SAT scores are exactly the same as Whites' scores.

1 2 3 4 5   4. I'm aware of racism, but I've never done anything racist personally, so let's not blame it all on me.

1 2 3 4 5   5. I don't have many friends who are from races other than my own, but I am making an effort to expand the diversity of my friendships.

1 2 3 4 5   6. When I find myself in a situation in which I am unfairly given advantages over people who are non-White, I reject those advantages.

1 2 3 4 5   7. Minorities make me nervous. There is a history of criminal behavior and aggressiveness that I'd rather avoid.

1 2 3 4 5   8. I would rather avoid the issue of racism than have someone confront me about it.

1 2 3 4 5   9. Examples of reverse discrimination, such as affirmative action, are a big problem for Whites in America.

1 2 3 4 5   10. Dominance over others is just a natural characteristic of White culture.

1 2 3 4 5   11. You can't just blame the media and politicians for racism. We all have to take responsibility for perpetuating it.

1 2 3 4 5   12. I prefer to live in diverse neighborhoods, work in diverse environments, and enjoy the fact that my friends come from all races and walks of life.

1 2 3 4 5   13. Most of the greatest artists and thinkers of the Western world have been White. My college courses have added people from other races to the curriculum, but it's just to make minority students feel included.

1 2 3 4 5   14. Yes, racism exists, but it's too complicated and overwhelming for me to deal with right now.

1 2 3 4 5   15. If we keep letting minorities into America from other countries, there won't be anything left of our great heritage.

1 2 3 4 5   16. If the media portrayed Black people more positively, racial tensions would end.

1 2 3 4 5   17. I think it's a good idea to take courses in college that expose you to other cultures, like courses in African-American literature or Chinese history.

1 2 3 4 5   18. I would feel completely comfortable dating and/or marrying outside of my race.

1 2 3 4 5   19. I consider myself to be colorblind. Race is completely unimportant to me.

1 2 3 4 5   20. I'm embarrassed about my racist upbringing and, as a result, I have a hard time dealing directly with racial minorities.

1 2 3 4 5   21. Racial minorities have brought many of their problems on themselves by relying on the welfare system and not making the effort to get a better education.

1 2 3 4 5   22. I think White people should help to end racism, which is why I usually vote for the Democrats.

1 2 3 4 5   23. If I really thought about it, I bet I could come up with plenty of examples of times I either made racist comments intentionally or unintentionally, or laughed at racist jokes, or took my racially privileged role for granted.

1 2 3 4 5   24. As a White person, I feel it is my responsibility to help eradicate racism and discrimination in our society.

1 2 3 4 5   25. It's just a fact that Asians are better at math and science than other groups and Blacks are more athletic than other groups.

1 2 3 4 5   26. Everyone is so politically correct these days that I'm afraid to open my mouth lest someone accuse me of being a racist.

1 2 3 4 5   27. Racism continues because minorities dwell on the past, like slavery and other things that happened a long time ago.

1 2 3 4 5   28. White people who live in the city or in other areas that are heavily populated by minorities should make a concerted effort to get along in their communities.

1 2 3 4 5   29. I would be comfortable with someone confronting me about racism if that confrontation would make me a better person.

1 2 3 4 5   30. Whenever I witness it, I confront people who make racist comments.

The following chart indicates which questions from the preceding list fit with each racial identity status. Those students who have identified themselves as White and completed the questionnaire are requested to put a check mark in the spaces in the chart next to each question to which they responded with a 1 (strongly agree) or 2 (agree). Although this exercise is not scientifically perfect, it should give those students who completed the questionnaire an indication as to where they fit on the White racial identity status model. The statuses under which they have put the most check marks indicate approximately where they fall in terms of racial identity status. Once the exercise has been completed, all students are asked to discuss the exercise. Revealing their racial identity status is the students' choice.

Contact		Disintegration		Reintegration		Pseudo-Independence		Immersion/Emersion		Autonomy	
1		2		3		4		5		6	
7		8		9		10		11		12	
13		14		15		16		17		18	
19		20		21		22		23		24	
25		26		27		28		29		30	

ETHNIC IDENTITY DEVELOPMENT

The Helms Racial Identity Development Model that was introduced in the preceding sections is not limited to racial development. It can also be adapted in terms of ethnicity. The Helms Racial Identity Model for People of Color describes the identity development of people in non-dominant groups in general. In turn, the Helms Racial Identity Model for White People describes the identity development of White people in relation to people from non-dominant groups in general. As with racial groups, ethnic groups must struggle to understand themselves in terms of their own group, the dominant group, and the relationship between the two. The following scenario illustrates how ethnic identity development parallels the racial identity development of people from racial minority groups.

Elizabeth's Experience

Elizabeth grew up knowing that she was Jewish and being moderately aware of her ethnicity and religion. However, even growing up in a large Jewish community, she did not understand her own ethnicity. She remained naïve and often celebrated the dominant religious holidays such as Christmas and Easter. Amidst Christmas presents and Easter eggs, she continued to say that she was Jewish without a real understanding of what that meant. At times, she devalued aspects about her religion such as kosher laws and going to synagogue. Although movies such as *Schindler's List* allowed her to connect with her heritage, these brief encounters only temporarily moved her into the Encounter stage.

She devalued her Jewish heritage until she moved to the Midwest and was no longer supported by a large Jewish community. There she was able to experience the difference between the dominant religion and her own religion. Somewhere between trying to explain that Hanukkah wrapping paper could not be red and green and struggling to find a synagogue with a young adult population, she began to enter the Immersion/Emersion stage. During the next year, she began to understand herself and find ways to appreciate other racial/ethnic/cultural groups as well as the dominant group. She struggled through the Internalization stage and had a few characteristics of the Integrative Awareness stage.

Fully immersed in an advanced multicultural course, she continued to learn about herself, her ethnicity, and other races, ethnicities, and cultures. However, another critical incident occurred in her second meeting with her White, male clinical supervisor as they discussed a new client who had been assigned to her. Elizabeth had not yet met the client and had only the client's name, undergraduate status (first-year student), and an anxiety diagnosis. The supervisor asked her to hypothesize why the client might be struggling with anxiety. Elizabeth remarked that she could not begin to make an educated guess, given the lack of information. Elizabeth remembers the supervisor stating, "Well, the client's last name sounds Jewish and she is a first-year student. The Jewish female culture has something called 'The Jewish American Princess.' It is likely that she has been mommy and daddy's little girl and now that she is away from her family, she does not know how to adjust. Her boyfriend might have broken up with her and she is feeling anxious."

Elizabeth sat in disbelief at the gross stereotypes that her well-respected supervisor was teaching. Not only did he minimize Jews and women, he also made the assumption that her client was heterosexual. She realized that he would easily think the same thing about her if he had known that she was Jewish. She spent the period between Rosh Hashanah and Yom Kippur (a period marked by introspection for Jewish individuals) deliberating about how to respond to her supervisor. At this point, Elizabeth was moving back into the Immersion/Emersion stage, valuing only her own ethnicity as a way to protect herself. As a new student, she did not feel that she had any allies in her department and had no one with whom she could discuss this situation. Thus, during a heated supervision session, Elizabeth inappropriately blurted out that she felt her supervisor was "anti-Semitic, misogynistic, and heterosexist."

Elizabeth remembered her supervisor calmly replying, "Does it make any difference to you that I raised a Jewish son?" She replied, "You can be Jewish yourself and anti-Semitic. The fact remains that you tried to teach me that being a "Jewish American Princess" was a viable component of the Jewish faith. How can I trust you to teach me anything about my other clients?" The session ended with Elizabeth walking out and going to seek help from her advisor. She remembers being advised to "work it out" with her supervisor. Elizabeth's semester evaluation stated that she "lacked professionalism," and this feedback was directly influenced by her relationship with her supervisor. Elizabeth spent the next two years in the Immersion/Emersion stage, until she was able to trust and connect with different faculty members. Neither ethnic nor racial identity development occurs in a linear fashion. Sometimes critical incidents can cause an individual to jump stages or return to earlier stages.

Ethnic Minority Identity Status Exercise

DIRECTIONS: Please examine the following questions, which are simply adapted from the questions in the Racial Minority Identity Status Exercise that was earlier in the chapter. Students who identify themselves as members of ethnic minority groups (Jewish, Nigerian, Pakistani, Italian American, Polish American, etc.) are requested to respond honestly to each question by circling the number beside each question that most closely corresponds to their opinion: 1 means "strongly agree," 2 means "agree," 3 means "neutral," 4 means "disagree,' and 5 means "strongly disagree." Students who do not identify themselves as ethnic minorities are asked to read through the questions in preparation for a group discussion.

1 2 3 4 5   1. Most of my friends are outside of my ethnic group.
                          I only have a few acquaintances from my own group.

1 2 3 4 5   2. Sometimes I think that my friends who are outside
                          of my ethnic group are not always supportive
                          about my ethnicity, but I don't have that many
                          friends within my own ethnic group either.

1 2 3 4 5   3. I am sick and tired of people who have problems
                          with celebrating ethnic diversity. I would prefer to
                          spend time with people from my own group.

1 2 3 4 5   4. I'm moving away from anger toward the oppres-
                          sors. It just isn't getting anyone anywhere.

1 2 3 4 5   5. I consider myself an activist, working with mem-
                          bers of all of the diverse groups in my community
                          to do away with racism, ethnocentrism, and other
                          forms of oppression.

1 2 3 4 5   6. The reason people in the dominant ethnic group are
                          successful in life is because they know how to work
                          the system to their advantage better than others.

1 2 3 4 5   7. I feel like a fish out of water. I can't say that I'm
                          happy about either my own ethnic community or the
                          prospect of moving into a neighborhood consisting of
                          mostly people from the dominant ethnic group.

1 2 3 4 5   8. I've never wasted my time hanging out with peo-
                          ple who are likely to look down on me because of
                          my ethnicity, and I'm not about to start now.

1 2 3 4 5   9. My friends from the dominant ethnic group are
                          very politically aware, so we manage to have pro-
                          ductive conversations about ethnicity, even if they
                          sometimes don't get my point of view.

1 2 3 4 5   10. I would be completely comfortable dating and
                          committing long-term to a person from the domi-
                          nant ethnic group.

1 2 3 4 5   11. My people need to stop whining and get beyond
                          how they are oppressed, because that's the
                          American way.

1 2 3 4 5   12. I think people pretty much determine their own
                          fate, with a little help from outside.

1 2 3 4 5   13. People from the dominant ethnicity listen to bland
                          music. There's no comparison between music that
                          comes from the soul and music that is just boring.

1 2 3 4 5   14. I didn't used to have any friends from the domi-
                          nant ethnic group, but I've made friends in college
                          with people from the dominant ethnicity with
                          whom I actually have a lot in common.

1 2 3 4 5   15. I'd prefer to live in a diverse community, where everyone just gets along.

1 2 3 4 5   16. I'm embarrassed that ethnic minorities are using the system by collecting welfare and unemployment checks.

1 2 3 4 5   17. People from the dominant ethnic group have caused a lot of problems for ethnic minorities, but now they have to deal with reverse discrimination and affirmative action, so I guess it evens out.

1 2 3 4 5   18. People from the dominant ethnic group may read books by Chaim Potok, go to Martin Scorsese movies, and eat at ethnic restaurants, but I think it's just lip service to prove they're not prejudiced.

1 2 3 4 5   19. I'm very confident about my ethnic identity now and can confront ethnocentrism firmly but without exploding in anger every time.

1 2 3 4 5   20. I am interested in either pursuing a career related to eliminating oppression and social problems, or if I end up doing something else, I definitely plan to give back to the community by volunteering or contributing in some other way.

1 2 3 4 5   21. Ethnicity isn't an issue with me. I prefer to just be viewed as a human being.

1 2 3 4 5   22. I'd like to start hanging out with more people from my own ethnic group, but I don't have the same interests as most people of my group.

1 2 3 4 5   23. I'm always surprised at how varied people of my ethnic group are.

1 2 3 4 5   24. People of my ethnic group are just as varied in their interests and outlooks as people from other groups. It takes all kinds.

1 2 3 4 5   25. Every person has a stake in making the world a better place for everyone.

The following chart indicates which questions from the preceding list fit with each ethnic identity status. Those students who have identified themselves as members of ethnic minorities and completed the questionnaire are requested to now put a check mark in the space in the chart next to each question to which they responded with a 1 (strongly agree) or 2 (agree). Although this exercise is not scientifically perfect, it should give those students who completed the questionnaire an indication as to where they fit on the ethnic identity status model. The statuses under which they have put the most check marks indicate approximately where they fall in terms of ethnic identity status. Once the exercise has been completed, all students are asked to discuss the exercise. Revealing their ethnic identity status is the students' choice.

Pre-encounter		Encounter		Immersion/ Emersion		Internalization		Integrative Awareness	
1		2		3		4		5	
6		7		8		9		10	
11		12		13		14		15	
16		17		18		19		20	
21		22		23		24		25	

CULTURAL IDENTITY DEVELOPMENT

As with racial and ethnic groups, those who fall into culturally non-dominant groups must also struggle to define themselves and their relationships with others. For instance, lesbian, gay, bisexual, and transgender people must negotiate identity development, and the same is true of people with disabilities.

Lesbian, Gay, Bisexual, and Transgender Identity Development

Lesbian and gay identity is different from racial and ethnic identity development in one primary way: Typically, an LGBT person's family is not part of the same group (in terms of sexual orientation or gender identity) as the LGBT person. This means that LGBT individuals must come to terms with their identity as lesbian, gay, bisexual, or transgender persons on their own and in a way that is quite different from members of racial and ethnic minority groups. There is no family group to help buffer the effects of **homophobia**, a strong negative reaction or fear of LGB individuals, **transphobia**, a strong negative reaction or fear of transgender individuals, or **heterosexism**, the perception that heterosexuality is the only appropriate and normal sexual orientation.

Considering the fact that LGBT individuals must "go it alone," it is understandable that such individuals often try to ignore their sexual orientation or gender identity in the first stage of LGB identity development, the **Confusion** stage (Cass, 1979). Although Cass's (1979) model was not originally written to include transgender individuals, the process of "coming

---

DEFINITION

Lesbian, Gay, and Bisexual (LGB) or *homosexual?* The term *homosexual* has fallen out of favor because of its association via the American Psychological Association between 1950 and 1973 as a psychological disorder. The terms *lesbian woman, gay man,* or *bisexual woman or man* are considered more empowering. The term *queer* has come into favor among some members of the LGBT community and the entertainment industry, but not all members of the LGBT community agree with the positive usage of a historically homophobic word.

DEFINITION

Transgender individuals' gender identity (man or woman) does not match their biological sex (male or female). Within the transgender community, there are additional subcommunities. For instance, *Cross Dressers* are individuals who feel more comfortable dressing in clothing (either partially, such as undergarments, or completely) of the opposite sex. This is different than someone who is a *Transvestite*, who dresses in the opposite sex's clothing for sexual purposes. *Transsexual* is often the term used for someone who would like to pursue sexual reassignment surgery (SRS) or knows that SRS would be appropriate. Many transgender people are aware that SRS would be appropriate for them, but choose not to pursue SRS because of financial limitations (cost of the surgery is often more than $50,000), concerns about medical complications, or personal choice. Choosing to not pursue SRS does not diminish their transsexual identity. *Drag queens* are men who dress in women's clothing. They may be transgender in their identity or simply performing. Identity is personal, and you will have to ask, rather than assume. At the time of this writing, there was not enough research on transgender identity development to present an identity model. Because of the various subcommunities involved with the transgender community, the term *GenderQueer* is growing in popularity. This term also acknowledges a political link with the LGB (queer) community.

---

out" in terms of gender identity often parallels the sexual orientation coming out process. During the initial confusion stage, lesbian, gay, bisexual, and transgender individuals often experience feelings of shame, anxiety, and isolation. After the **Comparison** stage, which is characterized by rationalizing same-sex feelings (e.g., "Maybe this is just temporary"), individuals enter the **Tolerance** stage. This is a critical stage where LGBT individuals are beginning to acknowledge their LGBT identity, but they do not necessarily accept it yet. Hence, individuals often say things like, "I'm gay, but not like those flamboyant gay people."

The **Acceptance** stage is characterized by LGBT individuals developing friendships with other LGBT individuals and accepting their sexual orientation. The **Pride** stage is when LGBT individuals become immersed in gay, lesbian, bi, and transgender subculture. Individuals in this stage may feel angry toward heterosexuals and may begin to feel free to break gender stereotypes and be "out" in public. Depending on personal experiences and the community, individuals may go out of their way to be visible or be LGBT advocates. When individuals make prejudicial statements about gay/lesbian/bi/transgender people "flaunting it," they are typically talking about LGBT persons who are in the pride stage. In the final stage, **Synthesis,** the individual's anger toward heterosexuals and heterosexual institutions (e.g., marriage) usually subsides and there is an acceptance of self and others.

For those students who identify as lesbian, gay, bisexual, transgender, queer, or questioning, college can be liberating and constricting at the same time. On one hand, being away from family obligations allows students to learn about their identity—especially their sexual identity. On the other hand, a great deal of social life on campus involves heterosexual dating. It can feel isolating to walk around campus and see programs dedicated to "Men, Women, and Relationships." Dating auctions, formal dances, even the assumptions in classrooms around marriage can remind LGBT people that they are on the outside of the college experience.

Max, one of the authors of this book, who has taught a course in multicultural counseling for many years, had not included LGBT persons as one of the special populations to be covered in his class. His definition of multiculturalism was limited to those groups the federal government referred to as the protected minorities (Black American, Hispanic American, Asian American, and Native American). The term *protected* means that these groups cannot fully participate in the American Dream without federal assistance. He argued that the LGBT population should not be included because there was insufficient time to cover such a major and significant topic. His compromise was to allow LGBT groups to be studied if they were members of one of the protected groups. Therefore, it was okay to study gay Asians or lesbian Hispanic Americans.

Max changed his view about including the LGBT population when an openly gay male gave a passionate speech at the end of one of his multicultural counseling courses. In his speech, the student stated that while he enjoyed the class, he felt he had been shut out because gay people experience the same isolation, rejection, and negative labeling that racial and ethnic minority individuals and groups experience. He pointed out that future counselors and teachers in public schools should understand LGBT identity development and how to treat students at various stages. In addition, he argued that counselors should create a school climate where LGBT people can grow and develop as heterosexual students do. Such teachers themselves must be clear about their attitudes and feelings toward LGBT people.

This student gave additional suggestions about what counselors can do, including:

- Having open dialogue about LGBT culture and history
- Offering LGBT support groups
- Having zero-tolerance policies against LGBT bashing
- Sponsoring LGBT appreciation and education programs

Max was so impressed by this student's articulate speech that he incorporated a major segment of his course to understanding and counseling LGBT clients. The response by students was overwhelmingly positive. At this point, he cannot imagine not covering the LGBT topic in his multicultural counseling course. This interaction highlights a key element in becoming multiculturally responsible—taking feedback as well as giving it!

Identity Development of People with Disabilities

As with LGBT people, we have defined persons with disabilities as a cultural group (that is, a group joined not by race or ethnicity, but through another commonality). However, the identity development of people with disabilities is much like that of members of racial and ethnic minorities.

Like racial and ethnic minorities, people with disabilities have been treated as second-class citizens by the majority culture because of their usually visible differences. Therefore, the identity development status of people with disabilities tends to be similar, beginning with a **Pre-encounter** phase, in which the person is aware of his or her disability but does not know other people with disabilities and is not informed about disability issues or the history of people with disabilities in America. This is followed by the **Encounter** phase, in which the person begins to confront his or her disability as an identity, and then the **Emersion/Immersion** phase, in which the person becomes deeply involved with disability issues/advocacy and socializes almost exclusively with other people with disabilities. In the **Internalization** phase the person moves away from defining himself or herself strictly in terms of the disability and begins to expand his or her circle of friends. Finally, in the **Internalization/ Commitment** phase, the person comes to view his or her disability as important but not as an all-encompassing part of his or her life (Leierer, Hunt, Brumfield, & Terminie, 2002).

DEFINITION

People with disabilities. The correct term to use is *people with disabilities* rather than *disabled people*, because people with disabilities prefer to be referred to as people first, not as if they themselves were the disability. In short, use "People first language." The term *handicapped* is no longer used.

RACIAL, ETHNIC, AND CULTURAL IDENTITY CONFLICTS: A SAMPLE ACTION PLAN

Students on college campuses deal with racial, ethnic, and cultural identity issues either consciously or unconsciously. It is reasonable to believe that the more racially diverse our campuses become, the greater our awareness of racial/ethnic/cultural identity becomes. For example, prior to desegregation, when Max's world was primarily Black, he rarely thought about race. He thought about race only when he encountered White people and people of other races. Max became keenly conscious of his racial identity as a Black man when he attended his first desegregated class in graduate school. He was the only Black student in a class of 25 and he felt alone, isolated, and lost, like a guest in a strange house.

While Max felt lost because he was accustomed to living in an all Black environment, there are Black students who feel anxious among other Black people because they were reared in mostly White neighborhoods. For example, Black students who attend Historically Black Colleges and Universities (HBCU) experience culture shock if they are not used to being among other Black students, Black faculty, and Black administrators. Many such students may never adjust to Black culture on college campuses and drop out to enroll in predominantly White colleges.

John's Experience

A few years ago, a Black man, named John, reported to a counselor in our university counseling center with a racial identity conflict. In essence, he was quite uncomfortable with other Black students and wanted to reduce his level of anxiety with them. John reported that he was extremely frightened when he attempted to walk through "the Set," a location on campus where a large number of African/Black-American and Latino(a)/Hispanic-American students hung out during lunch hour. John would take the long way home rather than walk through the Set, which was located at the center of campus. While John feared being among students on the Set, he was also excited, energized, and drawn to it.

In counseling, John told his counselor that he had been reared in a White neighborhood in a large city in the Northeast. His parents were both well educated and held positions in large companies, and made a combined salary of more than $300,000 per year. John's parents had always told him to avoid Black people and to socialize only with White people if he expected to be successful in life, and to avoid contact with Black people because they are very dangerous.

JOHN'S ACTION PLAN

John reported for counseling because he wanted to challenge some of the beliefs about Black people that his parents had instilled in him and he wanted to reduce some of his fears about them. The following is a treatment plan that the counselor used to help John to achieve his counseling goals.

First, the counselor invited John to participate in an action plan experience designed to help him learn, grow, and change with regard to understanding himself and the racial group to which he belonged. Having heard his story, the counselor convinced John that he understood why he could not connect with the Black community and saw Black people as inferior to White people. The counselor, who also happened to be an African-American man, believed it was important to accept John as he was rather than judge him based on his present perspective. Sometimes counselors of Color experience personal reactions to clients such as John who reject their own racial group.

Second, the counselor explained to John that the action plan was a tri-level action-oriented experience where he would move toward increased contact and involvement with Black people. He explained that Level One was observation (learning and growing from a safe distance), Level Two was investigation (learning and growing from a closer distance), and Level Three was direct participation (learning and growing from the closest distance).

To begin the process, the counselor asked John to assist in the development of the action plan by selecting experiences at each level with which he would be comfortable and could achieve his personal growth goal. The three levels and suggested ideas that the counselor and John worked out are explained in the following sections.

ACTION PLAN LEVEL ONE: OBSERVATION (LEARNING FROM A SAFE DISTANCE)

Check each item you believe will help you reach your goals and in which you feel comfortable participating.

1. Watch the films *School Daze, Do the Right Thing,* and *The Color Purple.*

2. Take a tour of two Black neighborhoods, one lower class and one middle/upper class.

3. Attend a Black church service.

4. Read three of the following books:
   a. *Three Negro Classics—Black Voices* by James W. Johnson
   b. *Sula* by Toni Morrison
   c. *Invisible Man* by Ralph Ellison
   d. *I Know Why the Caged Bird Sings* by Maya Angelou
   e. *Native Son* by Richard Wright
   f. *Passing* by Nella Larsen

5. Select a safe position on campus where you can observe what happens on "the Set."

6. Keep a personal journal of your reactions and feelings to each one of the preceding experiences. (These reactions and feelings from the journals were used as material and topics for discussion and exploration in the counseling sessions.)

ACTION PLAN LEVEL TWO: INVESTIGATION (LEARNING FROM A CLOSER DISTANCE)

Select from the following list each item that you believe you would feel comfortable participating in and that you believe would assist you in achieving your personal growth goals.

1. Interview selected Black faculty and staff members concerning their research interests to determine if you could get to know them better through their research and activities of mutual interest.

2. Talk with Black-American student leaders concerning their critical issues.

3. Interview your parents about the development of their attitudes about Black people.

4. Join a group of other Black students who share a pre-encounter racial identity status.

5. Continue to keep a journal of reactions and feelings generated from the preceding experiences to be used as topics for discussion in the counseling sessions.

ACTION PLAN LEVEL THREE: DIRECT PARTICIPATION (LEARNING FROM THE CLOSEST DISTANCE)

Select from the following list the items that are comfortable for you and offer the greatest opportunity for growth and change.

1. Build on the friendships you initiated in the investigation phase by arranging to have dinner with a Black person of your choice.

2. Volunteer to work on community service projects with a Black individual (e.g., mentoring Black schoolchildren, building a home through Habitat for Humanity, supervising recreation activities for youth).

3. Spend the weekend in the home of a Black person and observe his or her lifestyle, customs, traditions, family practices, roles of family members, needs, concerns, and issues.

4. Continue to keep a journal of reactions and feelings generated from the preceding experiences to be used as topics for discussion in the counseling sessions.

ANALYSIS OF JOHN'S ACTION PLAN

The counselor reported that in all of his many years of experiences as a multicultural counselor, his work with John was one of the most successful and rewarding. After six weeks of counseling, John's attitudes and behaviors toward Black people changed tremendously. In particular, he gained knowledge, reduced stereotypical views, and reduced the fear and anxiety he previously held. He was able to make new friends of Color, join an organization of African-American students, and spend time on "the Set" with his new friends. In addition, he was able to build friendships with other White students in his classes without becoming absorbed by their White culture. Due to his positive experiences with Black individuals, John moved from the conformity status to an internalization status.

Some of the following factors may account for these demonstrative changes:

1. The counselor accepted John as he found him rather than judging him as a "sell-out" or as an "Uncle Tom." In addition, John felt that the counselor genuinely wanted to help him and was invested in his well-being.

2. The novels and movies selected for John depicted Black people in a positive manner. For example, by reading Maya Angelou's novel *I Know Why the Caged Bird Sings*, John was able to understand some of the psychological consequences of growing up as a Black person in the 1940s in the Southwestern United States.

3. In touring poor Black neighborhoods, John learned two lessons about low socioeconomic level Black communities. First, many Black people sit on their front porches rather than stay inside their homes, because often the homes are not air-conditioned and residents find it to be cooler outside. Second, many Black men stand on street corners during the day, giving the appearance that they do not work or have jobs. To the contrary, John learned that many of these men hold evening or night jobs. These insights created **cognitive dissonance** because much of what he was learning was contrary to what he had been taught about Black people.

> ### DEFINITION
>
> ***Cognitive dissonance*** is when individuals feel conflicted, such as when they feel one way, but act in an opposite manner. This inconsistency often becomes so stressful that people change their minds or their actions to be congruent.

4. John's observations of Black students who clustered together on "The Set" paralleled a constant theme in Black literature, which is that Black people prefer group, collective, familial, and community settings rather than individual settings.

5. Through interviewing his parents about their family history and about their racial identity, John learned things about his parents he had not known before. He learned that they had migrated to Boston to find better jobs rather than work in the fields of Alabama. They were in complete denial about their history and wanted to forget the past and all of the people they had known. With regard to racial identity, they took a colorblind approach, believing that "people are people" and that the only race is the "human race." His parents added that their experiences with Black people had been characterized by pain and suffering while their experiences with Whites had been filled with comfort, peace, and prosperity.

6. It was through his participation in a Black male support group that John experienced the most relief. He learned in the first session that he was not the only Black person who was ashamed to be Black, who devalued Blackness and idealized Whiteness. John was relieved to learn that others had begun to question their previously held negative beliefs about Blackness and were in the process of transitioning into more positive attitudes. Through small-group discussion he observed that they had all come from similar backgrounds.

7. John developed a great deal of compassion and empathy for young Black boys and girls through a volunteer project located in a housing project in an extremely low-income section of the city. This project involved cleaning up the playground, repairing playground equipment, and teaching children how to be more responsible for their environment. Through involvement with these children, he became less judgmental toward poor Blacks. He pledged to assist at least two children toward achieving better lives when they grew up.

8. Through his volunteer work in the housing project, John met another college student (Jamal) who frequented "The Set," a place he feared more than any other place on campus. Jamal was a Muslim from the Midwest who was a member of a Black fraternity and a member of several Black organizations on campus. John and Jamal became instant friends, and the rest is history.

9. Overall, John learned a great deal about African-American history and how it has influenced the present condition of African Americans. His thirst to learn more about his own Black ancestry was amazing. He read all the books he could find, joined the Black Student Union, and expressed interest in becoming a member of one of the Black fraternities.

AWARENESS INTO ACTION: TAILORED ACTION PLANS FOR VARIOUS RACIAL/ ETHNIC/CULTURAL GROUPS

The benefit of creating an action plan for yourself is that it can be tailored specifically for you. Anyone can use the action plan format to build relationships with students, faculty, and administrators from different racial/ethnic/cultural groups. To help you get started with your action plan, consider beginning your observation phase with some of the movies and books in the following list. These movies present racial, ethnic, and cultural groups in both positive and negative ways. There is no movie or book that represents perfectly a group, because much diversity exists within groups. However, these movies and books typically show a current aspect of the group, a perceived aspect of a group, or past experiences of different groups. These movies and books should be viewed as starting points to examine various groups and open discussions with peers.

JEWISH PEOPLE

Movies: *Gentlemen's Agreement, Exodus, The Chosen, Schindler's List, School Ties*

Books: *How Jews Became White Folks* by Brodkin (nonfiction), *Sarah* by Orson Scott Card, *Ritual Bath* by Faye Kellerman, *Conversations with Rabbi Small* by Harry Kemelman, *Zaddik* by David Rosenbaum, *Night* by Elie Wiesel

CATHOLICS

Movies: *Shoes of a Fisherman, The Keys of the Kingdom, Boys Town, Becket*

Books: *Catholics and American Culture: Fulton Sheen, Dorothy Day, and the Notre Dame Football Team* (nonfiction) by Mark Stephen Massa

NATIVE AMERICANS

Movies: *Smoke Signals, Dance Me Outside, Lakota Woman: Siege at Wounded Knee, The Doe Boy, Thunderheart*

Books: *Storyteller* by Leslie Marmon Silko, *Love Medicine* by Louise Erdrich, *100 Native Americans Who Shaped American History* by Bonnie Juettner (nonfiction), *House Made of Dawn* by N. Scott Momaday

LATINO/HISPANIC AMERICANS

Movies: *My Family, Tortilla Soup, Stand and Deliver, Real Women Have Curves, Mi Vida Loca*

Books: *Last of the Menu Girls* by Denise Chavez, *Hunger for Memory* by Richard Rodriguez, *How the Garcia Girls Lost Their Accents* by Julia Alvarez, *Dreaming in Cuban* by Cristina Garcia

ASIAN AMERICANS

Movies: *Sayonara, The Joy Luck Club, Crash, Shogun, Tai-Pan, Noble House, Monsoon Wedding, Fire, Bend it like Beckham*

Books: *The Joy Luck Club* by Amy Tan, *Monkey Bridge* by Lan Cao, *The Woman Warrior: Memoirs of a Girlhood Among Ghosts* by Maxine Hong Kingston, *Eat a Bowl of Tea* by Louis Chu, *New X-Men #133* (comic book) by Van Sciver and Rapmund Morrison

AFRICAN/BLACK AMERICANS

Movies: *Roots, Crash, Higher Learning, Remember the Titans, Finding Forrester, John Q, Glory, The Color Purple, Do the Right Thing, Jungle Fever*

Books: *Uncle Tom's Cabin* by Harriet Beecher Stowe, *Life and Times of Frederick Douglass, Brothers and Sisters* by Bebe Moore Campbell, *What you Owe Me* by Bebe Moore Campbell, *Cane River* by Lalita Tademy

LESBIAN, GAY, AND BISEXUAL PEOPLE

Movies: *The Incredibly True Adventure of Two Girls in Love, But I'm a Cheerleader, Torch Song Trilogy, Chasing Amy, Kissing Jessica Stein, And the Band Played On, Fire, Go Fish, Tongues Untied, The L Word* (TV show), *Jeffrey, Broken Hearts Club, Saved*

Books: *Is it a choice?* by Eric Marcus, *Love, Ellen: A Mother/Daughter Journey* by Betty DeGeneres, *The Normal Heart* by Larry Kramer, *Vice Versa* by Marjorie Garber

TRANSGENDER PEOPLE

Movies: *TransAmerica, TransGeneration, Beautiful Boxer, Better than Chocolate, Different for Girls, Ma Vie en Rose (My Life in Pink), Boys Don't Cry, Ed Wood, The Adventures of Priscilla, Queen of the Desert, Stonewall, Paris is Burning*

Books: *Vested Interests* by Marjorie Garber, *Cross Dressing, Sex, and Gender* by Bullough and Bullough, *My Husband Wears my Clothes* by Peggy Rudd

EUROPEAN/WHITE AMERICANS

Movies: *I Remember Mama, To Sir with Love, American History X, White Lies, Breakfast Club, Crash*

Books: *Portrait of a Lady* by Henry James, *Ethan Frome* by Edith Wharton, *The Sound and the Fury* by William Faulkner

EUROPEAN AMERICAN/WHITE MEN

Movies: *Fight Club, Marty, Dead Poets Society, Pleasantville, Wall Street, Saving Private Ryan*

Books: "The Love Song of J. Alfred Prufrock" by T.S. Eliot, *The Grapes of Wrath* by John Steinbeck

EUROPEAN AMERICAN/WHITE WOMEN

Movies: *The Piano, The Hours, Woman of Substance, The Contender*

Books: *The Gate to Woman's Country* by Sherri Tepper

PEOPLE WITH DISABILITIES

Movies: *Charley, Miracle Worker, Finding Nemo, The Waterdance, Wait until Dark, What's Eating Gilbert Grape, If You Could See What I Hear, Children of a Lesser God, Ice Castles, Can You Feel Me Dancing?*

Books: *You Will Dream New Dreams: Inspiring Personal Stories by Parents of Children With Disabilities* by Klein et al.

Although these selected readings and movies are essentially leisure activities, the content is rich in history, culture, communication patterns, contemporary issues, and value differences. The purpose in reading these novels or watching these movies is to gain insight into the worlds of racially, ethnically, and culturally diverse groups. More specifically, this practice is another avenue for helping students, faculty, and administrators become multiculturally responsible on campus and in the real world. The insight gained and the personal growth experienced will be immeasurable.

CHAPTER AND PERSONAL REVIEW QUESTIONS

1. What is the definition of *racial identity*?

2. What are the five statuses of Helms's Racial Identity Model that people of color may express? What are the characteristics of each status?

3. What are the six statuses of Helms's Racial Identity Development Model that White people may express? What are the characteristics of each status?

4. Although Helms has not created a separate identity status model related to ethnicity, how can Helms's Racial Identity Model be applied to persons from various ethnic minority groups?

5. What are the six stages of Cass's LGBT identity development model and what are some of the characteristics of each stage?

6. What are the five stages of identity development for persons with disabilities and what are some of the characteristics of each stage?

7. At least one of the identity development models in this chapter will have applied directly to you. What was your identity status? Did more than one of the identity development models apply to you (e.g., racial and LGBT, or ethnic and persons with disability)? If so, what can you do to move ahead in two or more identity statuses at the same time?

8. What are the preferred terms used to describe the three cultural groups described in this chapter?

9. What is cognitive dissonance?

10. Has this chapter motivated you to create an action plan for yourself, based upon your current identity development status? Why or why not?

REFERENCES

Baldwin (1995). My dungeon shook: A letter to my nephew on the one hundredth anniversary of the emancipation. In *The fire next time*. New York, NY: Modern Library.

Cass, V. C. (1979). Homosexual identity formation: A theoretical model. *Journal of Homosexuality, 4,* 219–235.

DuBois, W. E. B. (1940). *Dusk of dawn*. New York, NY: Harcourt, Brace.

Helms, J. E. (1992). *A race is a nice thing to have: A guide to being a white person or understanding the white persons in your life*. Topeka, KS: Content Communications.

Helms, J. E. (1995). An update of Helms's White and People of Color racial identity
    models. In J. G. Ponerotto, J. M. Casas, L. A. Suzuki, & C. M. Alexander (Eds.),
    Handbook of multicultural counseling (pp. 181–198). Thousand Oaks, CA: Sage.
Helms, J. E., & Cook, D.A. (1999). *Using race in counseling and psychotherapy:
    Theory and practice.* Needham, MA: Allyn & Bacon.
Kivel, P. (2002). (Revised Ed.). *Uprooting racism: How white people can work
    for racial justice.* British Columbia, Canada: New Society Publishers.
Leierer, S. J., Hunt, B., Brumfield, K., & Terminie, M. (2002). *Disability issues.*
    Presentation at the American Counseling Association Annual Convention,
    New Orleans, LA., March 2007.
Woodson, C. G. (1933). *The Mis-education of the Negro.* Washington, DC: The
    Associated Publishers.

CHAPTER 3

▲▲▲
▼▼▼

Recognizing and Overcoming Privilege

BEFORE YOU READ

1. What is your definition of the word *privilege*? Does the term apply only to wealthy people or is there a broader definition? Please explain.

2. What are the different types of groups that might be privileged over other groups in contemporary American society? Describe each type of group and some of the ways they may be privileged over other people.

3. Do you think privilege is something you should accept or reject? Why?

INTRODUCTION

College is filled with unique experiences. For students of traditional college age, the college experience often means having more freedom, getting a credit card, making new friends, staying up as late as you like, eating whatever you like, going to parties, and taking road trips. For students who are older than the traditional age or students returning to college from the workforce, college can be unsettling and different from the workforce. Academically, colleges can provide open access to faculty and administrators, offer seemingly endless learning opportunities, and point you in the direction of either the career you have always wanted for yourself or the career you had not thought of before. As in the larger society, most colleges are explicit about their policies regarding respecting campus diversity and the

57

rights of all students. But before students believe that college environments are as free and protected as they could be, they should consider the following list of real incidents that have occurred on American college and university campuses in recent years:

1. At a large university, a Pentecostal preacher wandered around campus and asked students questions such as "Which is worse, a queer or a murderer?" Another day he said that the ERA (Equal Rights Amendment) stood for Eve Ruined Adam. Police asked him to leave for his own safety, rather than because he was breaking any laws.

2. A major national bank offered students T-shirts that read, "10 Reasons Why a Beer is Better than a Black Man" in exchange for applying for a credit card. Subsequently, the college chairman fired the firm handling their promotions and the college announced a solicitation ban.

3. A fraternity chapter organized a party where males dressed as GI's, and women dressed as Vietnamese prostitutes. Fraternity officials apologized.

4. A popular clothing manufacturer offered T-shirts that read, "Wong Brothers Laundry Service—Two Wongs Can Make It White" and depicted two smiling men with slanted eyes wearing conical hats. This triggered an e-mail and phone boycott of the company, which led to the shirts being removed from stores.

5. A costume company featured a costume mask named "Kung Fool" which featured buckteeth, slanted eyes, and a black eye from being beaten. After complaints, no more were distributed, but the manufacturer did not recall the masks. The company said that decision would be left up to the retail stores, but that they would accept returns.

6. Another costume company continues to sell a "Blind Referee Kit" which includes a referee jersey, dark sunglasses, and a blind person's walking stick.

7. University administrators disbanded a fraternity for having a party that featured guests wearing blackface. A picture from the party was posted online at a website. The picture had a fraternity member dressed up as a Ku Klux Klan member holding a noose over another student in blackface.

8. A sorority held a "Who Rides the Bus" party in 2001, where two members wore blackface and stuffed basketballs under their shirts to simulate pregnancy. About 1,000 students and faculty protested with a silent march.

9. The word *Spik* was found one morning spray painted on a building designed for Hispanic culture. At the time a Hispanic student was campaigning for student body president on a predominantly White campus.

10. In 2006, a fraternity publicized a "Halloween in the Hood" party that included a mock lynching (of a pirate) complete with fake gunshots in the background. The invitation encouraged partygoers to wear "regional clothing from our locale" such as "bling bling ice ice, grills," and "hoochie hoops." University officials responded by suspending any activities by the fraternity.

As you can tell, despite liberal, respectful college policies, there are many areas for growth in terms of multicultural responsibility on college campuses today.

Getting oriented to college life can also be challenging in less obvious ways than the preceding examples indicate. Many individuals who responded to our Internet survey stated that their first multicultural experiences occurred in college. Tanya, a White individual, said, "Growing up in a very racially homogeneous small town, I never had a conversation with someone from a race different from myself until college." Tanya went on to say that living with her roommate, who was Mexican American, was a good challenge for her. Lisa, a professor, stated that college was the first time that she had ever heard a foreign language outside of her high school Spanish class. Tarina, a biracial individual of African-American and Hispanic-American heritage, said that her first challenge was with her college roommate. She said, "We were always so proper around each other, never did anything together, although sometimes the offer was extended, but was never taken up on, and it just did not seem as though we related." Sharon, an African-American woman, stated, "I found that people of nonethnic backgrounds were truly oblivious to what happens in society as far as discrimination goes, although they try to understand."

> **REFLECTION**
>
> Although some people refer to White individuals as "nonethnic," remember from Chapter 2 that everyone has an ethnic background. White/European American is considered an ethnicity (e.g., Irish, Italian). However, White culture is not an ethnic minority. What are the implications of saying that White individuals do not have an ethnicity?

Diversity challenges on campus are not limited to White individuals and People of Color learning to live together, or even socialize with one another. Sometimes cultural challenges occur within a culture. Maria stated that although she is of Mexican and Peruvian heritage, she was raised in a primarily White environment. Her first challenge with diversity was when she interacted with other Latino(a)/Hispanic Americans on campus who did not understand her acculturation and wanted her to act like them. She said, "During my freshman year, I ran into many Latinos who were not 'colorblind.' Instead, they considered me not 'Latina enough.' I still do not understand those statements and choose not to accept their opinion of my integrated cultural beliefs and

REFLECTION

What were your first challenges with diversity on campus? How did you negotiate the situation? Were the results positive?

values." Jean, a Hispanic-American female, stated, "I identify myself as Hispanic, but do not 'look' Hispanic. The first challenge I had was as a freshman trying to convince someone of my Hispanic American background." Ellen, an Asian student, stated, "I'm really tired of people of color who are racist against other people of color. Most people feel that people of color can't be racist." As Ellen stated, anyone can be discriminatory. This can be a shock for a student who has grown up in a supportive and diverse environment. People tend to be drawn to people who are like them and find it easier to trust people who have similar traits, such as age and skin color. When college does not match this schema, and people of their own group are discriminatory, this can really shake students up.

While college can be an enlightening experience for people who have had little contact with diversity, it can be a different experience for those who are from diverse backgrounds. Theresa, who is Latina American and grew up in Miami, stated that her first challenge on campus was "feeling like a minority for the first time." Similarly, Rebeka stated that it was unusual for her to have to go to her classes on Yom Kippur, a high holy day of the Jewish culture, which involves complete fasting (no food or drink for 24 hours). Rebeka and others stated that an absence of sensitivity to the Jewish ethnicity was challenging. Nema, another Jewish woman, said, "I often found myself having to explain my cultural identity to my peers." It is important to remember that culture can be defined broadly to include ethnicity, religion, ability status, heritage, sexual orientation, gender, and socioeconomic status.

Other individuals talked about how sexual orientation was an initial challenge for them. Rob, a heterosexual male, stated that his first roommate in college was a gay man. Rob's roommate was open with his three roommates, but closeted to other people. "To witness his struggles for acceptance amidst rampant homophobia in the general learning environment was a significant learning lesson for me." Lisa, an African-American lesbian woman, said, "I live with triple jeopardy. I'm Black, female, and a lesbian. I barely talked to my first-year roommate because I was not prepared for any additional pressure in my life. I know that this isolated me from a potentially good friendship, but I had to take care of me." Transgender students often face additional struggles. Alexis stated, "Using the bathroom on the women's floor was difficult. I was starting to appear more masculine, and custodial staff told me that I needed to use the male bathroom. Although part of me was excited about "passing," I lived on the female floor and did not have access to a male or gender-neutral bathroom. I had no idea how to explain to custodial staff that I was a female to male transsexual."

The preceding examples illustrate that there are numerous challenges to overcome on college campuses in terms of multicultural responsibility. Particularly egregious and borderline illegal incidents occur. More often, the challenges are on a less dramatic, but no less important scale. This chapter will deal with some of the more frequently encountered challenges—in essence, those having to do with encountering and negotiating privilege on campus.

WHAT IS PRIVILEGE?

Consider this scenario, which illustrates racial privilege: Bandages are passed around to each student in a first-year humanities classroom. The instructor asks the students to raise their hands once the bandages are placed on the backs of their hands. The instructor reads aloud the label on the box, which says "blends with skin." But of course the bandages clash with many of the students' skin tones. The instructor explains that the closer a person's skin is to the color of the bandage, the more respect that person receives from the general public. The further a person is from the color of the bandage, the less respect that person is likely to encounter in his or her daily life.

The following list highlights some examples of **privilege** on a typical American college campus:

- The library is named after a White male, reminding students that they are attending a White college.

- Brochures about the campus are in English, and there is no mention of materials being made available in any other language, including Spanish or Braille.

- Social events conform to majority culture in that they focus strictly on heterosexual dating.

- Pizza parties are held on Friday evenings, paying no attention to the food/Sabbath restrictions of certain religious groups (Jews, Seventh Day Adventists, etc.).

- Courses focusing on racial, ethnic, and cultural groups (African-American literature, LGBT history, etc.) are considered "electives" rather than being core components of most degree requirements.

- A number of buildings on the campus are not easily accessed by students in wheelchairs.

- The food in the dining hall is representative of the majority culture ("ethnic food" consists of tacos, chicken chow mein, etc.).

- Cultural events such as films, special lectures, musical events, and theater are held in the evenings, meaning that only those students who either live on campus or are able to get to campus in the evenings are able to take advantage of these educational events.

- The football team's mascot is based on a Native-American stereotype of the brave red warrior.

As the previous examples show, privilege is about more than race. Privilege exists in terms of gender, sexual orientation, ethnicity, culture, physical ability, socioeconomic class, and religion. It may be true that the library is named after a White man because 30 years ago the college president was White, true that some of the buildings are very old and that making them wheelchair accessible would be difficult and expensive, and true that standard "American" meals such as baked chicken and meat loaf are easy and cost-effective to cook in mass quantities in school cafeterias. However, not talking about these examples of privilege allows privileged students to maintain their privileges and biases because they are not challenged to "see" other cultures.

Exercise for Recognizing Internalized Privilege

DIRECTIONS: Please read the following statements and visualize the people involved in each situation:

- The couple was caught by the resident assistant for cohabiting (i.e., spending the night together), which was against housing rules.
- The student activist decried the marked increase in campus date rape incidents.
- The student went to the instructor's office to ask for further direction regarding the term paper topic.
- The student finished class for the day and thought about how she would organize her evening.
- The student body president advocated for more common areas on campus.

Did you assume that the couple caught cohabiting were heterosexual? Did you assume that the student activist concerned about date rape was a woman and that the date rape incidents concerned only female victims? Did you assume that the student who went to the instructor's office walked right in, rather than possibly using a wheelchair or negotiating the area with a blind stick? Did you assume that the student who finished class thought about such matters as extracurricular activities, homework, and/or socializing, rather than about taking her child out of day care, preparing a meal for her children, doing her homework, arranging for a babysitter, and getting to her night job on time? Did you assume that the student body president was White and male? If you made any of these assumptions, then you have internalized the notion that certain groups are entitled to certain privileges: that to be in a couple is the domain of heterosexuals, that men do not really have to concern themselves with the realities of rape, that physically able people do not need to give access to a building a second thought, that all students are wealthy enough to afford to live on campus and not have to hold jobs at the same time, and that people who deserve to be in positions of prestige are White and male.

One characteristic of privilege is that people who have privileges are often unaware of their privileges. As the quotation from Newton Minow in the following box shows, those with privilege often accuse those without privilege of asking for "special rights," as if expecting equal rights were a way of avoiding real responsibility. The reality, however, is that those in the privileged groups are really the ones with "special rights" that others do not have.

There can be no doubt that some people in American society have more rights and privileges than others. When privilege is given to these

> ### QUOTATION
>
> *We've gotten to the point where everybody's got a right and nobody's got a responsibility.*
>
> NEWTON MINOW
> Past Chairman of the Federal Communications Commission

people because they are part of the dominant race, ethnicity, culture, gender, or class, those who are not part of the dominant group become extremely aware of privilege. Suddenly, they speak up to say they feel mistreated and ask for (or demand) equal treatment. Since college is a learning experience, should not awareness of other cultures be a major focus? Should not moving out of our collective comfort zone be part of the college experience?

It is easy for all of us to say that we do not agree with this privilege and that everyone should be considered equal. However, to move beyond privilege, we all need to do more than pay "lip service" to privilege; we need to actively resist it. To do that, we must recognize that even if we are members of diverse groups, we all benefit from privilege in some ways. For instance, all men, not just White men, benefit from gender privilege; all people who are

> ### REFLECTION
>
> How is your college encouraging majority privilege by maintaining the status quo? What can you do to change this?

not persons with disabilities benefit from ability privilege; and all hetero-sexuals benefit from sexual orientation privilege. No one is completely incapable of taking advantage of the privileges afforded them, unless that person is a member of every imaginable socially disadvantaged group. Although it may sound absurd, even comic in its over-the-top unfairness, un-less you are economically disadvantaged, a member of both an ethnic and a racial minority, and are a transgendered lesbian with a disability, you have some, if not many, privileges in contemporary American society.

TYPES OF PRIVILEGE

The following sections explore the various forms of privilege further, illus-trating privilege in terms of race/ethnicity, ability status, economic status, gender, and sexual orientation.

Racial and Ethnic Privilege

While most colleges are racially and ethnically integrated, students still remain segregated in many ways. Unfortunately, the racial and ethnic divide does not seem to be closing. This becomes clearer on campuses that offer large social organizations and clubs for their students. For example, one of the authors of this book recently asked members of a White fraternity about forming an al-liance with Black fraternities on campus. Members of one White fraternity said that the idea sounded good but that they could not see where the White fra-ternity would benefit. The White fraternity members said that they already had their fraternity house, a financially stable bank account, and great politi-cal connections, so they wondered what they had to gain via an alliance.

In an attempt to counter the arguments, the author pointed out that the White fraternity would gain several advantages by allying with Black frater-nities, including:

- the expansion of the perspectives of both the White and Black fra-ternity members,
- the acquisition by members of both the White and Black fraternities of inter-group communication skills, and
- the development of skills needed to live in an increasingly multicul-tural world.

However, though these benefits sounded noble, they were not powerful enough to change the attitudes of White fraternity members who did not want their comfort to be disturbed in order to connect with members of a Black fraternity.

These issues of racial and ethnic privilege exist across other social or-ganizations, and not only in the Greek system. For instance, campus Christian

groups often will not reach out
and ally with campus Jewish or
Muslim organizations, perhaps
out of the perceived notion that
Christian religions are dominant
in American society anyway, so
what would be gained other than

REFLECTION

How would you respond to the question,
"What can a minority student give a majority
student that he or she does not already have?

religious confusion by allying with other religious groups? Similarly, in most
U.S. colleges and universities, campus literary magazines and newspapers
tend to be staffed by mostly European-American students, who do not
actively solicit minority staff/contributions to these publications, perhaps
assuming—as reinforced by the mostly White U.S. publishing and news
industries—that literature and news are primarily the domain of White edi-
tors and writers. Lack of communication by student groups on university
and college campuses creates a racially and ethnically separatist attitude.

Unfortunately, these racially and ethnically separatist attitudes still domi-
nate college campuses. Such separation can be observed clearly in common
campus areas such as the cafeteria, where students of different races and ethnicities eat at separate tables; on fraternity and sorority row, where White fraternities and sororities are clearly differentiated from racial and ethnic minority
fraternities and sororities (if the ethnic minority Greek systems even have their
own houses); and even in classrooms, particularly humanities classrooms,
where students perceive that certain courses (e.g., African-American history)
are for one group and that certain courses (e.g., literature of Arab diasporas)
are for another group. Signs of racial privilege can be observed among the faculty and administration of many American colleges as well. For example, according to the Southern Poverty Law Center (*www.Tolerance.org*), minority
representation among full-time faculty members at American colleges and universities is only 13.9%. In addition, 88.6% of full professors at American colleges and universities are White. Clearly, the lines among racial groups are
sharply drawn. These lines need to be erased so that students have opportunities to expand their education to include contact and involvement with people from races and cultures different from their own.

Exercise for Recognizing Racial Privilege

In Chapter 2 we suggested using movies (and books) as a way to begin to raise
your multicultural responsibility index. Movies can also be used to increase
awareness of and thereby overcome internalized notions of racial and ethnic
privilege. View either in class or outside of class one or both of the following
films that focus on the African-American college experience. Both films are currently available on DVD.

- *Higher Learning* (1995, directed by John Singleton)
- *School Daze* (1988, directed by Spike Lee)

Pay close attention to the films as you watch, taking notes and considering the following questions:

1. If you watch *Higher Learning*, compare and contrast how the African-American and European-American students are or are not aware of and affected by racial and ethnic privilege on campus.

2. If you watch *School Daze*, which is set at a historically Black college, compare and contrast how the African-American students of different skin tones are or are not aware of and affected by racial privilege on campus.

Compare notes with your fellow class members and discuss your reactions.

Exercise for Recognizing Ethnic Privilege

As discussed in Chapter 1, race, ethnicity, and culture often cross over into one another. However, for the purposes of this exercise, think of ethnicity in terms of shared national ancestry, language, religion, or a combination of these traits. Mark with a check mark each of the following items that you think is an example of ethnic privilege.

_____ **1.** Most schools and offices are closed on national and state holidays. Christmas is also a national holiday, but no Jewish, Muslim, Hindi, or Buddhist holidays are national holidays in the United States.

_____ **2.** When a restaurant advertises that it specializes in "American food," the items on the menu are typically hamburgers, hot dogs, milkshakes, bacon and eggs, and apple pie. Restaurants that provide international foods such as souvlaki, pad thai, linguini, and sushi are not considered "American cuisine."

_____ **3.** Although all Americans who are not Native Americans immigrated to America at some point, more often than not, new immigrants from non-European countries (e.g., Mexicans, Arabs, Haitians, Cubans) have difficulty immigrating, whereas British, German, Italian, Greek, and other European immigrants enter the country comparatively easily.

_____ **4.** Despite the diversity of American culture, very few Hollywood films focus on the stories of people other than European Americans (usually Anglo Americans). Most films that focus on other ethnic groups are produced by independent studios, with the exception of Italian Americans, who are usually depicted as gangsters in crime dramas.

_____ **5.** Most of the top money earners in America are European-American males. We consider people like Donald Trump and David Geffen to be the "voices" of success and entrepreneurship in America. Rarely does anyone comment that Indra Nooyi (of East Indian descent) was named 2006's most powerful woman in business when PepsiCo Inc. promoted her to CEO.

_____ **6.** Although a large percentage of well-paid athletes are African American, nearly every team owner and coach in American sports is of European-American descent.

If you put a check mark next to all of the items in the list, you are correct. Note how ethnic privilege encompasses just about every aspect of American life: government, business, sports, entertainment, education, and cuisine.

Ability Privilege

In addition to racial and ethnic privilege, ability privilege clearly manifests itself on college and university campuses. While those of us who are not persons with disabilities notice our ability privilege, consider how such privilege can become painfully clear at an institution in a region where it snows. After the first ice storm, slips and falls leave college students in the position where they need to wear casts, use crutches, or sometimes even need the assistance of a wheelchair. These students quickly realize that their institutions are not physically available for them. Stairs are the most difficult access route for physically disabled persons to negotiate, yet they are typically the favored route into a building. To conform with federal regulations, most institutions have added access ramps, but they are often at the back of buildings. Aisles in libraries often are not wide enough to accommodate a wheelchair or crutches. These are just a few of many examples in which persons with disabilities must live with restricted access.

Furthermore, ability privilege goes beyond the physical structure of an institution. Consider how our ways of speaking tend to reflect unawareness of or disregard for people living with disabilities, such as "Stand up when your name is called," "Raise your hands," and "Do you see what I mean?" In addition, people continue to use catch phrases to tease each other, such as "Are you blind!?," or "Are you deaf?" Instructors often employ handouts or PowerPoint slides written in fonts that are difficult for students with visual impairments to read,

> **REFLECTION**
>
> Imagine spending a day walking around campus on crutches. Putting yourself in the position of a person with disabilities for just one day will not make you an expert on what it is like to have a disability, but it will help you understand the architectural limitations of your campus.

or speak too quickly for some people to physically take notes (such as students struggling with spinal cord injury), or require off-campus research that is difficult for students with disabilities to complete, as it may require significant off-campus travel.

Exercise for Exploring Ability Privilege

Although this exercise will not teach you what it is like to have a permanent disability, it can raise your awareness of the architectural limitations of your campus and the ways language privileges physical and mental ability over disability.

1. Research how well-equipped your campus is for students with hearing impairments. Does the institution provide any literature for hearing-impaired students regarding how to adapt to campus life and resources available to them on the campus? Are sign language interpreters readily available in classrooms, or are students expected to rely on lip reading? In the event of a fire or other emergency, are evacuation plans in place that speak directly to hearing-impaired students?

2. Participate in a trust walk. Have a classmate or a friend lead you blind-folded around campus. Take turns leading each other, and process your results.

3. Use a wheelchair or crutches throughout the day. Note whether or not wheelchair-accessible ramps are convenient or out of the way. When you talk to people not in wheelchairs, do they look you in the eye, or do they look at the top of your head?

4. Pay attention to your language and mark down in a notebook any situation in which you find yourself or others using language that assumes all people are mobile, have perfect vision and hearing, do not have any learning disabilities, and do not have any other physical or mental disabilities. Also note situations in which language is used to make fun of or look down upon physical and mental disabilities.

It is remarkable how unaware people are about disabilities, beyond the easily recognizable disabilities of blindness, deafness, and physical injuries that require the use of a wheelchair. There are less immediately recognizable physical disabilities such as spina bifida, cystic fibrosis, arthritis, scoliosis, multiple sclerosis, and Guillain-Barre syndrome. There are developmental disabilities such as dyslexia, learning disorders, and attention deficit disorder (ADD). Even though it is a viral disease, acquired immune deficiency syndrome (AIDS) is characterized as a disability because of the many permutations it can take. Again, privilege is not always about race and ethnicity, but about how the majority is unaware of individuals in minority positions.

> **REFLECTION**
>
> Consider how you would feel if you were working on a class project with someone who had one of the above-mentioned disabilities. Would the type of disability make a difference to your comfort level? Figure out if you have any biases toward the different types of groups and challenge yourself to figure out why you have these biases.

Economic Privilege

For many students, attending college is a natural progression in their lives. Their parents, grandparents, and maybe even great-grandparents attended the same college they are attending. By the time these students arrive on campus, housing, tuition, transportation, medical services, insurance, bank accounts, and other things essential for student functioning are already arranged. Such students need only to be concerned about academic performance and about extracurricular or self-enhancement concerns.

Another group of students is somewhat concerned about money. They attend college on a budget and may hold part-time jobs to pay for personal items. As crises happen in their families such as illness, unemployment, or divorce, these students may find it financially difficult, if not impossible, to attend school.

Finally, some students can attend college only with some kind of scholarship or financial aid package. Unfortunately, many of these students spend a great deal of their time worrying about their financial aid money, because it often does not come when they need it most. For instance, financial aid checks often are administered during the first two or three weeks of classes, which can make buying books in a timely manner difficult. Some international students may not receive their first paycheck for two months, in which case buying books, paying rent, and buying groceries may be delayed. In many cases, financial aid is not enough, and these students have to work full-time to survive. Not only do they work to support themselves, but they also may need to help their families back home. For instance, Carrie came to college from out of state, leaving behind her single mother with diabetes, a grandmother with Alzheimer's disease, and four younger siblings. Their father had abandoned them several years earlier. Carrie feels guilty being in college while her family struggles daily to make ends meet. She has a scholarship but has to work two extra jobs to pay for housing, food, and books. Often, she is too tired to study after her second job, but she needs the money to survive.

Obviously, economic status makes a big difference in how students experience college. To further complicate matters, wealth privilege (or lack thereof) is linked with race/ethnicity privilege, gender privilege, ability status privilege, and other privileges. For instance, when you picture people within each of the economic statuses listed in the beginning paragraphs of this section, do you envision different races or cultures? Was the highly privileged group White? Did you notice a gender split? Which group did you imagine would be the smartest? Have you ever heard someone say, "I am fine with Black people, just not poor Blacks," or, "She's going to have to act more masculine if she wants to compete with me in the corporate world"? Statements like these show just how deeply we in America equate economic status with White male privilege.

For these reasons, it is important to recognize not only how some students are privileged by their wealth, but also how students from diverse backgrounds are often lumped into the category of "poor" or "lower class," even when they may not be. For example, Henry, an African-American son of a well-established medical doctor, was labeled by his college as needing special assistance when he in fact did not. He was placed on the minority-mentoring program to help minority students succeed academically, personally, and socially. Henry needed no such help. He had graduated from high school with a strong "A" average in the hard sciences and mathematics. In addition to his college administration's assumption that he needed extra help, he was asked in his physics class if he had made a mistake in his course selection. After convincing the professor that he was indeed in the right place, he proceeded to do excellent work and made one of the highest grades in the course. Henry did not need financial assistance since his father was one of the most successful medical doctors in their city. Simply because he was African American he carried the stigma of being financially needy and academically deficient.

Economic privilege manifests itself in still other ways, such as when students try so hard to fit in economically that they end up putting themselves in financially perilous positions. For instance, many college students take pride in their image, especially as it relates to the latest styles and fashions in clothes. Some students may put special emphasis on their appearance to avoid the stigma attached to being on financial aid. Concern over image also may come from one's racial, ethnic, or cultural background, such as the cultural value among Latino(a)/Hispanic Americans called *que diran*, which means, "making a good impression," or the Asian-American version of making a favorable impression called *saving face.*

The bottom line to remember is that not every student on campus is on equal footing financially. Furthermore, recognize that, though wealth may be disproportionately in the hands of European-American men in American society, not every White student has money in his or her pocket, and not every minority student is on financial aid. Challenge your stereotypes about money as it relates to race, ethnicity, culture, and gender.

Exercise for Negotiating Economic Privilege

DIRECTIONS: Read the following scenario and rank order your responses from 1 to 5, with 5 meaning the most multiculturally responsible and 1 meaning the least multiculturally responsible.

During a small-group discussion about computers, Tanya (a White student) mentions that she began using a computer when she was five years old, which is why she feels comfortable taking tests online. Brad (an African-American male) responds by saying, "It must've been nice to have a computer when you were young." Tanya responds by:

_____ Remaining silent

_____ Asking Brad, "Did I offend you?"

_____ Saying, "I am simply stating something about my life."

_____ Exploring Brad's response by saying, "Seems like you are saying I should be ashamed of my past. Am I misunderstanding you?"

_____ Responding positively, "Yeah, it was nice. I was very fortunate. That's why I go out of my way to help others who need assistance with computers."

Pick the response that you feel is the most multiculturally responsible for you. After you have rank ordered them, please break into small groups to discuss why you chose your rankings. Remember that most of the answers involve subtle differences that will be more or less attractive answers based on personal differences. In addition, discuss the risks involved with each response. You will learn more about becoming multiculturally responsible from listening to others and their preferences. There is no right answer, so please focus on *why* people choose a particular response. After the small-group discussion, please return to the large group and report what you learned in your small-group discussion.

Gender Privilege

Gender privilege, that is male privilege, exists in many different facets of campus life just as it does in American society, where studies continue to show that women do not earn as much as men for the same work, where stereotypes of women as emotionally driven, irrational beings still persist, and where the physical objectification of women in advertising and other media is still the norm.

Jean Kilbourne, author of *Can't Buy My Love: How Advertising Changes the Way We Think and Feel* and the documentary *Killing Us Softly*, poignantly emphasizes the way the media industry exploits women. Although some media images may portray women as being powerful, these same advertisements often subtly subvert women. For instance, many advertisements show only parts of a woman's body, often deleting the eyes or the entire face. Examples are the Disaronno liquor advertisement showing a woman's lips and an ice cube, or the close-up of a woman's behind in black panties and black lace tights that is advertising hairspray (BedHead products). Women in advertisements tend to be leaning on men or facing away from the camera, while men's bodies are shown in their entirety and facing the camera. Other more damaging media images are violent or dehumanizing toward women, such as those that show women in cages (e.g., Bebe, Diesel) or restrained, such as the Nintendo Game Boy Pocket advertisement which features no information about the gaming system but instead shows a woman tied up on a bed. Advertisements also demean femininity in general, such as the Amstel Light Beer advertisement that says, "Think of it as a light beer that's not in touch with its feminine side" or the Alpha Omega watch advertisement that says, "Almost as complicated as a woman. Except it's on time."

Aside from media, gender privilege strongly exists within the American education system. Gender privilege often begins during elementary school, where teachers respond differently to girls and boys in the classroom. Overall, boys are more likely to be corrected, criticized, praised, and helped. The nature of teacher feedback also differs based on gender. Boys are criticized for behavior problems and praised for intellectual accomplishments, while girls are criticized for lack of ability/low intellectual performance and praised for effort, cooperation, and dependent behaviors (Dweck & Elliott, 1983; Sadker & Sadker, 1994). The result is that women learn to doubt their ability, but behave well in the classroom. Unfortunately, unless college professors are acutely aware of gender and language styles, they may inadvertently respond differently to female and male students. For instance, in conversations, men tend to talk for longer periods than women do and are more likely to interrupt when someone else is talking. As such, during a discussion in a college course, it may appear that men have more of a "voice." One example of how male privilege exists in campus life is the Greek system, in which often men are afforded fraternity houses while women either are not afforded sorority houses or are only afforded space within residence houses. On other campuses, sororities are not allowed to possess alcohol in their living environments, whereas fraternities are allowed to possess alcohol.

REFLECTION

Think about some of the ways you (whether you are male or female) participate in male privilege. If you are a male student, do you take advantage of your privileged status? If you are a female student, do you sometimes defer to male privilege to avoid being "difficult"?

Another example of male privilege on campus manifests itself in language. Consider the use of the word *freshman*. This term is an artifact of an era when only men were allowed entrance into higher education. As a result, many schools are changing their wording to be more inclusive of women, by using the term *first-year students* instead of *freshmen*."

Exercise for Recognizing Male Privilege

Spend a day noting situations on campus in which men seem to have a privileged status over women. You should consider all types of situations. For instance, does your instructor attempt to balance coverage of writers of both genders in your literature class? How many people attend men's sports events and how many attend women's sports events (and do they seem to be equally funded)? How many fraternities are there and how many sororities (if your campus includes a Greek system)? Is the fraternity housing better than the sorority housing? Which housing is more convenient to campus? Are women equally represented in campus organizations such as the radio station and the newspaper? Do women hold prominent positions (such as president, director, etc.) in these organizations? Compare your notes with those of other students.

Heterosexual Privilege

People who are lesbian, gay, or bisexual tend to receive less respect than heterosexuals in U.S. society. A campus climate study (Rankin, 2003) revealed that one third of gay college students had reported harassment in the previous year. Half of these students said that they hid their sexual orientation to avoid intimidation, and another fifth feared for their physical safety. Furthermore, 43% described their campus as homophobic. The study also stated, "While most colleges publicly commit to creating a welcoming and inclusive environment, their actions and policies do not support these goals."

Why do lesbian, gay, and bisexual students experience harassment and/or hide their sexual orientation from others? Because as in American society as a whole, where in many states lesbian, gay, and bisexual people can still be fired from their jobs simply for being homosexual, where gay couples are not afforded the same rights as heterosexual couples (such as inheritance and hospital visitation rights), and where people are assumed to be heterosexual unless proven otherwise, heterosexuals hold a privileged position on college campuses.

Consider, for example, how many colleges and universities still do not include sexual orientation as a protected status in campus policy because lesbian, gay, and bisexual people are not recognized at the state or federal level as a protected group. Does your college infirmary or health service center allow same-sex partners to receive health services or are services available only to spouses? Even if many colleges and universities do protect lesbian, gay, and bisexual students via campus policy, the environment of all campuses still privileges heterosexuality over homosexuality. For instance, how many homosexual couples would dare to hold hands walking across campus, while heterosexual couples routinely do?

> **REFLECTION**
>
> Think about ways in which you privilege heterosexuality in your daily campus life. When you attend a campus dance (unless sponsored by the LGBT student group), do you automatically assume that the dance will consist entirely of heterosexual couples? Do you assume that the famous writers you study in your literature class or the influential historical figures you study in your history class are or were all heterosexuals?

Exercise for Recognizing Sexual Orientation Privilege

DIRECTIONS: Please break into small groups and respond to the following questions:

    1. Recall one experience or encounter with a person whose sexual orientation was different from your own. If you are lesbian, gay, or bisexual, obviously that is your daily experience, so narrow it down to a single memorable encounter in which your sexuality or the sexuality of the other person was relevant. How would you evaluate the way you handled the situation? If you are heterosexual, did you adopt an attitude of superiority/condescension toward the lesbian, gay, or bisexual person? Why or why not? If you are lesbian, gay, or bisexual, did you find that in that situation you deferred to heterosexual privilege or defied it? Please explain.

2. In what ways in your daily campus life are you aware of or blind to the existence of lesbian, gay, and bisexual students, faculty, or staff? How often are you exposed to lesbian, gay, or bisexual issues on campus (campus newspaper coverage, special events, classroom discussion, etc.)?

Gender Identity Privilege

Gender identity is a relatively new (at least in terms of visibility) and confusing topic for most people because it encompasses issues of gender and somewhat overlaps with issues of sexual orientation. Some students, who are transgender, experience incongruence between their sex (male or female) and their gender (man or woman) (Israel & Tarver, 1997). All people have a gender/sex relationship (some congruent and some incongruent) and all people have a sexual orientation, but gender identity is significantly different from sexual orientation. In addition to those who feel a incongruence between sex and gender, some other transgender individuals feel that both genders coexist within themselves (this may in fact be true; the number of infants born with both sexual organs is more than most of us realize, with a choice and a surgical procedure typically made very shortly after the baby is born) and often choose to describe themselves with the term *two spirited*. More recently, the term *genderqueer* has gained in popularity to encompass the range of people who are questioning or are completely sure of the incongruence of their own gender and sex. Regardless, transgender students are at a disadvantage in terms of both gender privilege (they do not benefit from male privilege because they are perceived as neither male nor female) and sexual orientation privilege (they do not benefit from heterosexual privilege, because they are perceived as being lesbian, gay, or bisexual, regardless of personal identification).

The issue of gender identity can become confusing for administration and students when it comes to room assignments. Imagine Menna, who is a new student on campus and identifies with a congruent identity: both female (sex) and a woman (gender). Her roommate, Lindsay, however, is a female by birth but internally identifies as Garrett, a man. Gender identity is not connected to sexual orientation, although Menna may be concerned because she is naïve about transgender issues. Administration is likely to struggle because they do not know where to place "Garrett."

Students and administrators at some colleges have found some interesting solutions. Wesleyan University in Connecticut, a liberal arts college founded by Methodist Church leaders, began a program in 2003 that allowed students to be assigned to a "gender-blind" floor in residence life. This floor is reserved for students requesting to be matched with a roommate without the consideration of gender (College dorm, 2003).

Going even further, Smith College in Massachusetts opted to remove gender language from their constitution (Girls college dumps pronoun, 2003). Smith College is an all-women's college, and students wanted to show support for their transgender colleagues who are uncomfortable with female pronouns. The administration stated that they would continue to accept only women, but they would not reject students who undergo sexual reassignment surgery (SRS) while they are students. Therefore, if Suzy undergoes SRS during her time at Smith, she would graduate as Steve—thereby allowing an all-women's college to graduate men. Despite these complications, the school appears to be invested in being multicultural. The director of the institute of diversity told reporters, "Smith College is a college for women, and within that there is a place for all kinds of women."

But these are rare instances. Most people, and certainly most colleges and universities, have not yet attempted to accommodate transgender students in any way, either because they continue to value gender (and perceived sexual orientation) privileged norms, or because they are confused about how to handle the situation, or both.

> **REFLECTION**
>
> If you are not a transgender person, have you ever met anyone who is? How did you view that person? Did you take the privileged position that the transgender person was "confused" or "misguided"? Did you assume the person was lesbian, gay, or bisexual, even though sexual orientation does not typically have anything to do with transgender concerns? Why or why not? If you are lesbian, gay, or bisexual, how do you view transgender persons? Do you embrace their concerns or do you reject them because they cloud the issue of sexual orientation?

Exercise for Recognizing Gender Identity Privilege

To get an idea of how important the distinction of gender roles (and consequently gender itself) are in American society, browse through the Sunday newspaper and look at the arts, culture, and fashion sections, as well as the advertising throughout the paper. Or look through a current magazine that deals with popular culture such as a men's magazine (*Details, Maxim, Men's Health*), a women's magazine (*Allure, Mademoiselle, Vogue*), or general pop culture magazine like (*Us* or *People*). Think a little more deeply about gender than you ordinarily might when flipping through such a newspaper or magazine. What are the things that American culture values about gender? What is it that makes a woman a "real" woman and a man a "real" man according to the depictions in advertising and pop culture? In what ways are people depicted as being rewarded for fulfilling the ideals of their gender?

AWARENESS INTO ACTION: OVERCOMING PRIVILEGE

Many students first encounter diversity in their new home in a college residence hall or apartment building. Students quickly become aware of their
own feelings of privilege when they find themselves living among both men
and women, and in the same room with people from different races,
ethnicities, sexual orientations, and gender identities.

Exercise for Overcoming Privilege: Circle of Significant People in Your Life

(Adapted from Parker, Archer, Scott, 1992)

Survey the significant people in your life and see if the following characteristics
are included:

_____ Persons with physical disabilities

_____ Persons with learning disabilities

_____ Lesbian women, gay men, and bisexual women and men

_____ Transgendered persons

_____ Asians or Asian Americans

_____ Latino(a)s/Hispanics or Latino(a)s/Hispanic Americans

_____ Native Americans

_____ European Americans

_____ Senior citizens

_____ Arabs or Arab Americans

_____ Biracial or multiracial people

_____ Economically disadvantaged people

_____ Persons with wealth

_____ Muslims

_____ Catholics

_____ Mormons

_____ Jewish people

_____ Africans or African Americans

_____ Indians or Indian Americans

DIRECTIONS: Place a check mark (✓) on the line beside each individual you believe is included within your circle of significant people (not including parents or relatives). Then place a double check mark (✓✓) on the line beside individuals not included but whom you would like to include. Now explain your choices and include your reasons for not selecting some individuals from the list. Why are some people in your circle of significant people and some are not? Do you privilege certain people over others? Try overcoming this by making a concerted effort to get to know someone outside of your circle. This is one way to recognize the value of other people and overcome your privileges.

Growth toward overcoming one's sense of privilege tends to involve a fair amount of introspection. Introspection, which means thinking about something deeply, usually takes a great deal of time and energy. Given enough energy and time, individuals can begin to learn to appreciate and honor their own and other groups. However, energy and time are often in short supply when it comes to roommates. Students will evaluate each other quickly and decide if they can trust one another. Sometimes, without knowing, students will offend each other without even saying a word. In general, roommates must balance creating enough room for their own culture without overpowering others. Without talking about these issues, there is likely to be an imbalance, which will feel *like* one of you has privilege and the other one does not have privilege. Furthermore, students need to be prepared for complicated issues and treat fellow students with the respect and dignity they deserve.

Sometimes the best way to learn about other people and to overcome privilege is to go back to the basics: break bread together. Maybe it needs to be white bread, marbled bread, pumpernickel bread, tortillas, or even rice—but eating together is a nonthreatening way to appreciate each other.

While breaking bread seems too simplistic to include as a mechanism for change, it is a life experience that is universal; everybody eats regardless of racial, ethnic, and cultural differences. Therefore to facilitate intercultural relations, people might try sharing a meal that is reflective of the many backgrounds of those in attendance. One such example is a cross-cultural exchange feast (CCEF) created by students. The CCEF could exist in many forms. Two student groups could co-sponsor the event and have their group members bring traditional foods and spend time mingling with one another and learning about each other's backgrounds. Another form would be to have students enrolled in a diversity course (or another course) bring in food or organize an outside event where they can focus on each other's identities.

The CCEF can consist of a variety of foods representing the many groups on campus and feature music and activities that also speak to groups that would not typically be represented by food, such students with a disability or LGBT identity.

The CCEF would be wrapped up by short speeches from the president of the student body, a faculty representative, and/or the president of the college. All speeches would focus on the role of diversity in college, making the point that a college is made stronger by its multicultural makeup and that a college becomes even stronger when students, faculty, and administrators from various races, ethnicities, and cultures come to know and appreciate people with different hues and different perspectives.

CHAPTER AND PERSONAL REVIEW QUESTIONS

1. What is the definition of *privilege*?

2. What is racial and ethnic privilege, and what are some of the ways it manifests itself on college campuses?

3. What is ability privilege, and what are some of the ways it manifests itself on college campuses?

4. What is economic privilege, and what are some of the ways it manifests itself on college campuses?

5. What is gender privilege, and what are some of the ways it manifests itself on college campuses?

6. What is heterosexual privilege, and what are some of the ways it manifests itself on college campuses?

7. What is gender identity privilege, and what are some of the ways it manifests itself on college campuses?

8. What other types of privilege exist that have not been covered in depth in this chapter? Are thin people privileged over average weight or overweight people? Are people who are physically attractive privileged over people who are average looking or perhaps not physically attractive? Please elaborate.

9. What are some of the ways to overcome privilege?

10. Now that you are more aware of privileges, are you motivated to give up or overcome your privileges for the sake of the greater good? Why or why not?

REFERENCES

Dweck, C., & Elliott, E. S. (1983). Achievement motivation. In P. Mussen (Ed.), *Handbook of child psychology, Vol. IV: Socialization, personality, and social development.* New York: Wiley.

College Dorm 2003: Sex Doesn't Matter. (2003). *WorldNetDaily.* Retrieved February 8, 2005, from http://www.worldnetdaily.com/news/article.asp?ARTICLE-ID=32741.

Girls' college dumps pronoun "she": Students want it to be place "for all kinds of women." (2003). *WorldNetDaily.* Retrieved February 8, 2005, from http://www.worldnetdaily.com/news/article.asp?ARTICLE_ID=32742.

Israel, G. E., & Tarver, D. E. (1997). *Transgendered care: Recommended guidelines, practical information, and personal accounts.* Philadelphia, PA: Temple University Press.

Parker, W., Archer J., & Scott, J. (1992). *Multicultural relations on campus: A personal growth approach.* Philadelphia, PA: Accelerated Development.

Rankin, S. R. (2003). Campus climate for gay, lesbian, bisexual, and transgender people: A national perspective. The Policy Institute of the National Gay and Lesbian Task Force. Retrieved February 8, 2005, from http://www.thetas force.org/downloads/CampusClimate.pdf.

Sadker, M., & Sadker, D. (1994). *Failing at fairness.* New York: Charles Scribner & Son.

▲▲▲
▼▼▼

CHAPTER 4

Racial, Ethnic, Cultural, and Gender Variables in the Classroom

BEFORE YOU READ

1. What were your expectations about the college classroom experience when you attended your first classes? Did you expect to fit in regarding your instructors' expectations of punctuality, attendance, classroom participation, and interaction with the instructor? Why or why not? In what ways have you found that you are attuned to these classroom expectations and in what ways have you found that you are not attuned to these expectations?

2. Have you ever felt that the instructor or other students unintentionally insulted or minimized you by their use of racist, ethnocentric, homophobic, sexist, or otherwise denigrating language? If so, how?

3. Have you ever felt that the instructor singled you out to be the representative of your race, ethnicity, culture, or gender? If so, how? Have you ever felt that the instructor silenced you from speaking based on your race, ethnicity, culture, or gender?

4. Have you ever been assigned a textbook that excluded or minimized the importance of your race, ethnicity, culture, or gender to the subject at hand? If so, did the instructor supplement the textbook with more inclusive in-class or hand-out information?

5. Have you ever run across blatant prejudice, discrimination, or stereotyping on the part of your instructor, directed either at you or at someone else in the class? If so, what, if anything, did you do about it?

INTRODUCTION

Academic classes typically evoke thoughts of buying new textbooks and school supplies, understanding class content and completing homework assignments, waking up early and getting to class on time, participating and interacting with other students and the instructor in class, and so on. What students less often consider when thinking about the college or university academics, however, is that not all students experience the particulars of academic life in the same way.

THE VARIABLES OF ACADEMIC LIFE

In some cases, colleges may reflect the values of the dominant race, ethnicity, culture, or gender, and these values may clash with the individual values of many students. As such, the classroom can inadvertently seem to reject the values of many individuals. Consider how some students might feel if a class syllabus included the following notes and guidelines:

- Students should attend all classes and be on time for class or their grades will be adversely affected.

- Students are expected to participate actively in class by interacting with the instructor as an equal participant in the learning process, asking questions aloud in class, and shouting out responses during classroom brainstorming sessions.

- The instructor for this course is old-fashioned. Please don't take it personally when the instructor occasionally uses "politically incorrect" language, as no offense is meant by it.

- At times during this class, we will focus on issues of diversity. Those students representing appropriate diverse groups are encouraged to speak up and share their views. At other times, the class will focus on the typically recognized "great thinkers" of this discipline, at which time the instructor will ask other class members to speak up.

- The instructor has chosen to use a popular textbook that was originally published in 1961 and has proved successful through 15 editions. This textbook provides the typical positive view of U.S. society that we are all used to, without too much focus on the negative.

Although general rules are necessary to carry out the learning process, how might some students feel about the preceding set of guidelines? Each student in a diverse classroom will come from a different racial, ethnic, cultural, and/or gender background and may not be able to or desire to accommodate to the preceding guidelines for various reasons, which will be examined in more detail later in this chapter. The particular variables pointed out by the example guidelines are those related to punctuality and attendance, classroom participation and interaction with the instructor, classroom language, being singled out or silenced in the classroom, textbook bias, and blatant bias/discrimination in the classroom.

Academic Variable #1: Punctuality and Attendance

Punctuality and attendance are issues that differ greatly from country to country and within U.S. society. For example, students raised in Europe or White U.S. society often learn that it is important to not only show up, but to show up slightly early for an appointment or for a class. In addition, appointments typically are scheduled in advance and confirmed. In Japan, attendance is expected, and there is no such thing as being "fashionably late." Rather, lateness is interpreted as being incredibly rude. However, Malaysian and Indonesian individuals are not as concerned about being on time, unless the individual is Chinese Malaysian, in which case promptness is very important. You did not assume that everyone labeled as Asian would have the same standards of attendance and punctuality, did you?

The point here is that concepts of attendance and punctuality are not universal. These things are viewed differently by people from different cultures. For those who were raised with European-American values, negative assumptions are often made about people who "blow off" class or "stroll" in late for a class or appointment, assuming that lateness means disrespect. As a student, you cannot change the views of your instructor or those of other students, but you do have control over your assumptions about those who attend or do not attend class and about those who arrive late or show up on time. Becoming more aware of how your culture may clash with the college culture or how you view students whose concepts of attendance and punctuality differ from your own will assist you in becoming an MRP (multiculturally responsible person).

> **REFLECTION**
>
> Which cultures might benefit from a lecture style of teaching? Which cultures might benefit from a more informal, discussion type of academic setting?

Exercise for Recognizing Attendance and Punctuality Variables

It would be a mistake to ask you to observe the attendance and punctuality of students in your various classes and then make generalizations based on who tends to show up regularly and on time and who does not. Your observations might lead to cultural stereotypes based on one individual's actions. Instead, go to the Internet and read about standards regarding time and attendance in different cultures across the world and accepted practices among various racial, ethnic, and cultural groups in the United States. Keep in mind that just because there may be certain standards based on national origin and racial/ethnic/ cultural group, it does not mean these practices are set in stone and practiced by all members of those groups. Some may have adjusted to the expectations of their current location, whereas some may have been raised in a way that contradicts the overarching values of their group. As with all things, keep an open mind, but remember that different people have different standards regarding punctuality and attendance.

Academic Variable #2: Classroom Participation and Interaction with the Instructor

Another variable in academia is how students are expected to participate in the classroom, which ties in with how students should interact with instructors. Some classrooms are set up in a lecture style, in which students are expected primarily to concentrate on taking notes and the instructor often appears to be unapproachable. Other classrooms tend to encourage questions, discussion, and in general a more interactive format, including working closely with the instructor inside and outside of class. Israeli children are taught to correct an instructor when they feel the instructor is saying something incorrect, whereas Vietnamese children are taught to be quiet unless called upon to recite memorized material. When asked what was the most recent challenge with diversity in his academic situation, Roberto, a 54-year-old Mexican-American male, responded to our Internet survey with the following comment:

> I felt that the instructors from the majority culture did not understand my culture sufficiently to offer insights into my clinical training, and in fact I was misunderstood by faculty. For example, my respect for instructors was misinterpreted as passivity.

As the preceding examples illustrate, some people may interpret silence as respect, while others interpret it as disinterest. Additionally, some people may interpret vociferousness as appropriate, while others interpret it as loud or overly aggressive behavior. In keeping with the focus of multicultural responsibility, we suggest that you educate others around you—including your instructor—when you expect that your culture's values regarding classroom interaction may be misinterpreted. For instance, Jennifer, one of this book's authors, remembers a first therapy session with a Native-American client. The client began the session by saying, "It is part of my culture to avoid eye contact. I often will attempt to have eye contact, but if I naturally look down it is not because I disrespect you or that I am lying." This openness and awareness of impact helped both individuals work together, and translates readily to an academic situation in which a student might be open about such matters with his or her instructor.

International students may find classrooms particularly challenging if the American college classroom is their first contact with American society. Aside from trying to learn the language, learning how to buy books, and negotiating the parking or bus system, these students are expected to quickly adapt to the rules of the classroom. International students are sometimes confused by the shifting classroom culture (i.e., classroom participation rules differ from instructor to instructor). As such, if you know that this aspect of your culture is likely to be misinterpreted, then we encourage you to inform your instructors privately if you are uncomfortable speaking up in class or if you find that you seem to be irritating the instructor or other students by being vociferous. Most instructors will be interested to learn about your culture and will appreciate that you have made an effort to fit into the classroom situation. Conversely, if you are confused about someone else's classroom behavior, then inquire politely about her or his behavior without making assumptions. The process of providing and seeking information about cultural differences is an important part of being an MRP.

Exercise for Recognizing Classroom Participation and Instructor Interaction Variables

As noted in the previous section's exercise, it would be a mistake to think that you can become attuned to understanding these variables by simply observing students in your classes and making racial, ethnic, and cultural generalizations based on those observations of a few people. Some students from groups in which speaking up and interacting with instructors is commonplace may actually be shy, and conversely some students from groups in which attentive silence is appreciated may have assertive personalities and like to participate and interact regularly. Still others from groups customarily more docile may have learned to adjust to their current situation, while those from groups customarily more vociferous may have adjusted accordingly. Generalizations never work, but to get a better idea of how different cultures perceive participation and interaction differently, go to the Internet and research how participation and interaction (not just in classroom situations but in any group or mentoring situation) is commonly viewed in different countries of the world and within different racial, ethnic, and cultural groups within the United States. You may find that there are a lot more variations than you think.

Academic Variable #3: Classroom Language

Cultural values are often transmitted through language. Although one of the classroom guidelines in the first section was overt (for the purpose of illustration) about the instructor being "old fashioned" and occasionally guilty of political incorrectness, usually instructors who use insensitive language are not aware of it.

The most insidious and frequent example of insensitive classroom language occurs when an instructor (or another student) refers to male students as "guys," but refers to female students as "girls," which diminishes the maturity and power of female students. Part of the problem is with the English language itself. Students often complain that the word "woman" does not feel appropriate, as it labels college-age females in a way that makes them seem older than they actually are. Yet, college-age females are certainly no longer "girls" either, and an age-neutral term that would be the equivalent to *guy* does not exist (the term *gal* might be the equivalent, but it is seen as an antiquated term). In other words, the language for women seems to be polarized (a female must be viewed as either a little girl or a fully grown woman) while the language for men is a gradient. We suggest that instructors and students alike get past their notion that "woman" or "man" are words reserved for people beyond college age and accept that by the time people graduate from high school, they deserve the adult designation as "women" and "men."

Another situation in which instructors and students alike might unconsciously diminish other students through the use of language is when the terms *dark* or *black* are used in a context meaning "evil" or "bad" (e.g., "The evil dictator had a black heart," or the like). Such meanings are not lost on students of color, who are fully aware that such language has been used to discredit persons of color by equating skin tone with criminal motivations.

> **QUOTATION**
>
> *If thought corrupts language, language can also corrupt thought.*
>
> GEORGE ORWELL

Language, especially colloquial terms, is powerful and is sometimes, either consciously or unconsciously, used against certain people. For example, the term *Indian giver*, means someone who gives a gift and then takes it back. It is surprising that this term continues to exist, given that most people are aware that the Native-American people had their land stolen and were subjected to germ warfare (Loewen, 1996), yet this term is typically used in a humorous context. Another example of offensive language is the term *paddy wagon*, which refers to the police vehicle that collects drunken people. What many people may or may not realize is that the word *paddy* is an Irish slur and the term *paddy wagon* reinforces the stereotype that Irish people drink too much. Another example of offensive language is the term *going Dutch* on a date, which is actually a term created a century ago as a slur toward the Dutch, implying that the Dutch were too cheap to pay for another person's meal. Still another term often used without understanding the context is *rule of thumb*, meaning "a basic guideline to follow"; it may surprise many people to know that the phrase is derived from Colonial American life, indicating that men were allowed to beat their wives, but only with a stick as wide as or narrower than the thumb. Other common phrases that we may not realize are racially, ethnically, or culturally offensive include *yellow bellied, Irish flu, dark continent,* and *white lie.* When such terms are used either by an instructor or by other students in the classroom situation, the classroom becomes a place in which not all students feel welcomed into the academic environment.

On the plus side, language also has the power to empower and enlighten in a classroom context. For instance, when an instructor or other students demonstrate an awareness of the origins of such negative phrases by calling attention to them, or when an instructor or other students show their sensitivity to diverse groups by using currently accepted terminology for various racial, ethnic, and cultural groups, as well as for women, then the academic classroom becomes a welcoming environment. Although terms such as *Chinese American* or *Colombian American* may feel wordy, using these terms helps everyone in the classroom environment recognize the value of different groups that continue to contribute to American culture as a whole. The ability to reconstruct language is powerful and allows people to acknowledge diversity through spoken and written word.

REFLECTION

What are other terms that may be offensive to people? Speak up the next time you hear these terms.

DEFINITION

Some currently accepted terms not defined previously in this book include **sexual orientation,** which is used in place of the out-of-date term *sexual preference* and demonstrates an awareness that sexuality is not a choice, and **cultural mosaic,** which is now used instead of the term *melting pot,* because a mosaic more accurately represents how each diverse group in American society adds to the whole picture without losing its own character.

Exercise for Recognizing Language Variables

This exercise is more conducive for a group than for individuals because it involves awareness of terms, phrases, and characterizations with which some people might not be familiar. Please work with other classmates to compile a list of terms/phrases/characterizations for each of the following groups that might be used innocently in a classroom situation but that might make women and students from certain racial, ethnic, and cultural groups feel stereotyped, minimized, or otherwise insulted. Keep the list in mind and try to avoid these terms/phrases/characterizations (as well as those discussed in the preceding paragraphs) in the future.

Women:

_____

People from specific countries of the world/Ethnic groups in America (e.g., Brazilians/Brazilian Americans, Swedish/Swedish Americans):

_____

Africans/African Americans/Black people:

_____

Europeans/European Americans/White people:

_____

Asians/Asian Americans:

_____

Hispanics/Hispanic Americans:

_____

Native Americans:

_____

LGBT people:

_____

Arabs/Arab Americans:

_____

Indians/Indian Americans:

_____

Economically disadvantaged people:

_____

Middle-class people:

_____

Wealthy people:

_____

People with disabilities (physical or mental):

_____

Protestants:

_____

Catholics:

_____

Jewish people:

_____

Muslims:

_____

People of other religious affiliations (Hindi, Buddhist, Jehovah's Witness, Seventh Day Adventist, etc.):

_____

Academic Variable #4: Being Singled Out or Being Silenced

Instructors probably would not overtly ask students, in their course guidelines, to speak up as representatives of their racial group, ethnic group, cultural group, or gender. Nor would an instructor be likely to directly ask students to silence themselves. Nonetheless, we included these scenarios in one of the sample course guidelines at the beginning of this section to illustrate the point that these types of situations frequently occur in classrooms all across America. Typically, singling out and/or silencing students occur without any intentional malice on the part of the instructor. Yet, situations like these are further ways in which some college students may find that the academic experience is not the same for everyone, that sometimes certain variables may need to be addressed to level the playing field.

Imagine this scenario: During a discussion on the Holocaust, an instructor asks a student wearing a Star of David (a Jewish symbol) if he had family killed at the death camps. The instructor asks the student to speak about how this has affected him and his family. Is this interaction acceptable? If the answer is not obvious, then try this scenario: During a discussion of the Civil War, an instructor asks the one African-American person in the classroom to talk about how slavery has affected her and her family. What's wrong with this interaction?

Something happens in groups, including classrooms, in which there is not much diversity: Those in the minority are sometimes called upon to speak for their entire group. This phenomenon occurs across the spectrum: for instance, in women's studies classes in which only one to two men are enrolled, or in history classes in which few women or few racial, cultural, or ethnic minority individuals are enrolled. Being called on to speak for your group depends on the composition of the group. However, racial minorities are disproportionately called on to speak for people of color. There are two negative outcomes from this phenomenon.

First, it forces the individual singled out into a position in which his or her response can create positive or negative judgments of their entire group amongst the other students in the classroom. Speaking for one's group denies the speaker individuality and moves him or her outside of the "mainstream" of the class. Singled-out students in a classroom setting might nonetheless reply because of pressure, or because they lack the confidence to say, "I am uncomfortable speaking for my entire racial/ethnic/cultural group."

Second, it could shut down the critical thinking process. Hearing the perspective of the singled out student, other students may come to believe that they "know" the minority perspective when they really only know one minority person's perspective. For instance, if Bob, an African-American man, tells the classroom that he has never felt directly affected by the legacy of slavery in any way, does that mean no African-American person has? To think so would involve using very flawed logic. One person's perspective does not constitute a consensus.

We encourage you, as a student, to be aware when you are hearing only one voice. If you notice that one person is being called on to speak for an entire group, remember that one or two voices do not represent the perspective of an entire group. By asking your instructor for additional resources such as books or videos, you are inviting the instructor to broaden the syllabus without piling on too much extra work.

The opposite of being singled out in the classroom is having no voice at all, or being silenced. For example, research has shown that instructors tend to interrupt women more than men. In addition, instructors tend to call on men more than women. In essence, women often do not have a voice in the classroom. Other students, such as those from racial, ethnic, or cultural minorities, may feel that they are silenced insofar as they are asked to provide minority perspectives but are either not called upon or are not taken seriously when they speak up about course content as a whole.

> **REFLECTION**
>
> How are your classrooms set up? Are men called on more than women? Is the classroom culture inviting for racial minorities? International students?

Whether the situation involves being singled out or being silenced, students may find that they feel intimidated about giving instructors crucial feedback about these matters. If students are aware of inequities in classrooms and do not feel comfortable speaking directly with their instructors about these matters, students should look into alternative way to deal with the situation. Some campuses may be equipped with a person in the position of ombudsman—that is, an individual assigned to address student needs and concerns in a confidential manner who investigates complaints, reports findings, helps students negotiate with instructors, or simply consults with students. Other campuses may not have hired someone into the specific position of ombudsman, but there may be other ways to deal with such matters. They should be outlined in your campus policies and procedures book or on the college website, or students can find out about how to handle such situations by speaking with their advisors.

Exercise for Recognizing Singling Out and Silencing

Be careful not to misinterpret singling out and silencing and turn your genuine concerns into instructor witch hunts. Some situations that look like singling out or silencing may be exactly that, while other situations that look like singling out or silencing may not actually turn out to be what you think. Be careful not to assume. Just because an instructor likes to go around the room and put students on the spot does not mean the instructor is singling out an African-American student when he or she asks the student to comment on the topic at hand, which happens to be related to African-American experience. And just because an instructor cuts a student short doesn't necessarily mean the instructor is purposefully cutting the student off because of the student's race, ethnicity, culture, or gender. The student might just be off the point. Singling out is the act of purposely and publicly making students feel on the spot specifically because of their race, ethnicity, culture, or gender. Silencing is the act of purposely and publicly shutting students up because of their race, ethnicity, culture, or gender. With this in mind, learn more about singling out and silencing by holding a group discussion. Without naming names, students could share their experiences (or lack thereof, which might make for an interesting counterpoint). This group exercise is a quick and easy way to brainstorm examples and decide as a group what situations are clearly cases of singling out and silencing and what situations are borderline or not really cases of singling out and silencing.

Academic Variable #5: Bias and Lack of Diversity in Textbooks

Though this is perhaps a more common problem in elementary and high school textbooks, which must be approved by often conservative state and district textbook selection committees, college textbooks are nonetheless still capable of favoring the majority perspective and merely paying "lip service" to multiculturalism and gender balance. Often there persists a sense that textbooks to a degree remain "whitewashed," or scrubbed clean of potentially controversial facts about certain important individuals or mentions of particularly ugly points in American history so that majority individuals do not need to feel challenged on their long-held views about these individuals or historical moments. James Loewen begins his book *Lies My Teacher Told Me* with the example of Helen Keller, who is important in American educational history because she was able to learn to read and write despite being blind and deaf. Few people know, however, that Helen Keller was a radical socialist and that she spoke out forcefully about how blindness was concentrated in the lower social classes. This is because often textbooks do not want to appear to be advocating "non-mainstream" political views, such

---

REFLECTION

Does material in your textbooks appear to be one-sided? Is material presented from a diverse perspective?

---

as those Keller held. Rather, they prefer to focus on Keller as an individual who overcame adversity and leave out the controversial material.

Other facts often left out of American history textbooks include the fact that President Woodrow Wilson was involved with the KKK, that Thomas Jefferson owned 267 slaves and only freed eight (all of whom were his blood relatives), and that, despite his reputation as an emancipator, Abraham Lincoln was quoted as saying, "I am not, nor ever have

---

REFLECTION

Continue to examine points in American history that might be less than savory. Look up President Andrew Jackson and his involvement with the Trail of Tears or President Franklin Roosevelt and his involvement with Japanese-American internment.

---

been in favor of bringing about the social and political equality of the white and black races" (cited in Loewen, 1996).

All of this is not to say that textbooks, particularly American history textbooks, ought to make a point of negating everything positive about famous American individuals, nor that they ought to focus exclusively on ugly points in American history. Rather, it is to say that textbooks should not try to "clean up" history to make it more palatable. Doing so creates an inaccurate portrait of an extremely complex and varied history, and we do not gain a deep understanding of history when certain important facts are simply left out of the picture. The fact is, however, that many textbooks and courses, especially those related to American culture, tend to be watered down. Books tend to erase important facts that complicate our history in important ways. The result is that American heroes appear like gods and goddesses rather than like sometimes flawed individuals, which all people are. Many of us have become so used to the idea of American heroes as untouchable heroic figures that when the details of their lives reflect racist or sexist attitudes, instructors and students do not know how to process this information. However, if American history were told accurately, then as a culture (or a classroom) people could see the faults of those who lived before them and strive to do better. To become an MRP, individuals are encouraged to remain open and willing to hear the whole truth about America and its history. Part of the whole truth is that there are some wonderful aspects about American culture, the strongest of which is the idea of freedom. So, rather than feeling ashamed about some aspects

REFLECTION

Can you graduate having studied only
White/Western thought? If yes, what is the
impact of that? What does this say about your
college's commitment to diversity?

of America's past, it is important for everyone to seek the truth with open eyes and recognize that American culture is still evolving.

Students do not always respond similarly to textbook content, whether it is "watered down" or not. If a textbook does state the facts about less than positive aspects of American history, White students often feel blamed for society's wrongs. This especially happens during discussions on slavery and White privilege. Often students will raise their hands and say, "I did not own slaves so do not blame me" or "There's nothing I can do about my privilege, it's just given to me." Clearly there is no easy answer about how to "correct" slavery or "modify" White privilege. However, as stated in Chapter 3, it is each person's responsibility to be aware of his or her privilege and power, and minimize how he or she contributes to an oppressive system.

When discussing a popular book on counseling individuals from a diversity perspective, graduate students on a public listserv responded with differing opinions. Brad, a 29-year-old European-American graduate student, stated, "When I took the course, I felt that I should be apologizing for being White. I would not recommend this book." Cathleen, a 33 year-old European-American graduate student, disagreed and said:

> I for one felt that the discomfort I experienced while reading the text, and while taking part in discussions, led to some very useful soul-searching and questioning of ideas I'd taken for granted for years. I'm not sure that the goal of teaching human diversity classes should be discomfort—but I'm not sure the goal should be keeping everyone comfortable, either. This is not an easy topic. I applaud anyone involved in motivating others to look within themselves, no matter which text is used.

Tamala, a 27-year-old African-American graduate student, added:

> I do not think that discomfort is a bad thing at all. In fact, if people are honestly and richly exploring and discussing issues of multiculturalism and diversity, then I would be afraid if people all walked away with warm and fuzzy feelings about ourselves and others. These are tough issues in which people are required to look at their own history with privilege and oppression, both from a personal and historical standpoint. . . . While I don't think it's necessarily fruitful for a particular group to be vilified, I also don't think it's fruitful to rescue people from uncomfortable feelings brought up by such discussions.

With such differing views on what discussions should be brought into the classroom, it's no wonder that some instructors play it safe by toning down diversity (and consequently uncomplimentary instruction about the majority culture) in their classrooms. Unfortunately, toning down information often does not allow students to see the full picture of our society and it does not teach students to appreciate diversity. Even though you may have a strong reaction while reading this book, we encourage you to continue to read, despite any discomfort you might feel. Having your comfort disturbed often parallels opportunities for personal growth and change.

Even if a textbook does do a good job of avoiding whitewashing, there are a limited number of topics that can be covered in a classroom within a quarter or semester. It may seem that topics of diversity are glossed over or that only one diverse group's experience is examined in any detail. To enable students to deepen their understanding of the subject matter, instructors will often have students do projects or term papers that encourage exploring a topic in depth. These papers and projects allow good opportunities for students to learn about their own or others' race, culture, ethnicity, or gender as it relates to the class topic. For instance, as part of her anthropology assignment, Marcia, a part-Native-American student, wanted to learn more about the Native-American side of herself. She began her self-exploration experience by interviewing her parents about her family background. Having learned that she was part Blackfoot, she read all the literature she could find about her tribe. Finally, Marcia made arrangements to visit an Indian reservation where Blackfoot Indians lived. During her visit, she was told stories about her tribe from the elders that were consistent with what her parents had told her and with what she had read. Marcia declared that this experience was one of the most valuable learning experiences in all of her college studies.

You may feel that you are not enrolled in a class that allows you to study topics from a diversity perspective. You may be assigned topics such as depression, music history, Joseph Conrad, or theater appreciation, and wonder how those topics might relate to diversity. But once you put some thought into it, the ideas should begin to make themselves apparent. For instance, papers and projects on these topics could focus on depression among Nigerian-American women, musical themes in common between European classical music composer Franz Schubert and African-American jazz composer Miles Davis, homoerotic images in Conrad's *Heart of Darkness*, or the similarities between themes in Greek playwright Euripides' plays and current Cuban culture.

Exercise for Recognizing Bias and Diversity in Textbooks

Go back and look at a few of your course books from a previous semester, particularly books for humanities courses such as history, sociology, literature, art history, and music appreciation (math and science, by nature, are not courses that lend themselves to topics of diversity). How diverse are these books? Keep in mind that some courses are expected to be more diverse than others. A course on nineteenth-century European philosophy is not going to feature much, if any, material about women and members of diverse racial, ethnic, and cultural groups. However, an introductory textbook in any given humanities subject should strive to present a diverse and varied perspective, particularly any history or sociology textbook and any textbook devoted to arts and literature (especially twentieth-century) when women and people from all backgrounds began to find themselves in the position to have their art shown, plays performed, literary works published, and music appreciated. If certain groups were under-represented in the textbook, did the textbook author point out that this was because certain groups did not have opportunities at the time or place discussed?

Academic Variable #6: Blatant Instructor/Faculty Bias and Discrimination

Not listed as an example in this section's opening course guidelines as a variable students experience in academia is blatant discrimination, because obviously no instructor would call attention to his or her biases on a syllabus. In this day and age, however, blatant discrimination on the part of instructors and other faculty does still occur, if much less frequently than it once did, even with checks and balances in place at most colleges and universities to prevent and/or deal with such occurrences. As in the larger American society, bias and discrimination are not problems that have been "solved," and so they can carry into academia just as they can carry into any other part of American society. Unfortunately, there are still instructors and other faculty who believe that there is not a place for women and African Americans in the fields of math and science (and, in contrast, there are those who believe that Asian-American students should *only* be enrolled in math and science); there are still those who refuse to acknowledge that lesbian, gay, and bisexual individuals have a place in American society and therefore in the classroom; and there are still those who believe that certain racial, cultural, and ethnic populations simply are not college material.

No instructors or other faculty today are going to be totally open about their blatant biases and risk losing their jobs. However, such biases may be felt by students nonetheless in less blatant ways, ways that may be hard to prove and may go unchallenged. Earlier in this book, we mentioned a student who spent considerable time convincing his instructor that he, as a Black man, did in fact belong in his physics class. Though the instructor was not blatant and did not make any racist comments directly to his face, the student nonetheless became aware that the instructor was much harder on him than he was with other students—in a way that did not challenge him to do better but seemed clearly designed to frustrate him to the point of dropping the class. In addition, the instructor consistently acted in a manner, both when the student spoke in class and when the student met with the instructor during his office hours, that clearly indicated that the instructor did not take the student seriously. At one point the instructor even asked the student, "Do you really think you're cut out to take physics?," when in fact the student comprehended the material quite clearly and typically scored as well as other students on quizzes.

This example is, we hope, a rare experience. Unfortunately, these situations do occur, and when they do, students may become locked into stereotypes about themselves when they are trying to complete a course and may end up doing poorly when they find it's easier to give up than to challenge assumptions about their place in academia. The far-reaching effects of such bias are that students may end up not pursuing their life goals, and may even change majors to avoid the discomfort of being discriminated against. Students in the majority can afford to simply attend class, study, and not be encumbered with the psychological distress brought about from bias and discrimination. Consider another example, from Celia, an African-American female student, which we learned of via our Internet survey:

> The university experience is liberating, challenging, and exciting, but the orientation leader did not mention that I would be tested on other matters outside of the classroom. In my early semesters at the university I had high anticipation for my academic future. This enthusiasm faded with time when I began to feel isolated from my classmates because I was one of the few minorities in my upper level science courses. It is not easy to cope with these types of problems in academics; moreover, it is difficult to survive instructors that believe I should have been "weeded out" when I took the prerequisite classes. I often thought to myself, "Is this the universal attitude toward all students that approach their instructors for help, or is this because I am a Black woman?" I believed the latter was true. Regrettably, this would not be the only incident that tested my self-esteem. While visiting an instructor for clarification concerning a chapter, he stated, "If you can't understand the principles of biochemistry from my lecture, then I suggest you seek academic counseling because there is nothing I can do for you. Frankly, I am surprised you made it this far in my course." These words shook me to my core and lowered my self-esteem. I wondered how I could succeed in a predominantly White university system where there was not a strong support for minorities. It was comforting for me to know that I was not the only student trying to survive these racial barricades. I made friends with other students, particularly minorities, in my courses. I even joined a club for minorities in science. We formed an alliance, aiming to be the strongest students academically in our classes, regardless of the lingering voices of discouragement.
>
> For other students who are facing some of the academic challenges I encountered, I would suggest turning these negative experiences into sources of empowerment. I had to become proactive. I sought out all possible sources to help support my academics. You must to keep knocking on all doors until you are able to get answers and support you need to survive.

Finally, White students can help change the academic culture by continuing to be inviting to students outside their race. We can learn from those who are different from us culturally because they have different worldviews and customs. By reaching outside of our comfort zone to other races, and realizing that education is not a vicious competition, we can begin to change some of the racial tension and distrust that plagues so many college campuses.

What else can you, as a student, do if faced with these "isms" in the classroom? First, walk into the classroom believing that you have an opportunity to learn, and know that, like every other student, you earned your place to take any course in the college. Second, notice occurrences of blatant bias and discrimination, if they exist in your particular classroom situation. Third, if such occurrences persist, seek help in ways outlined by campus policies and procedures, because there is no reason you should tolerate them. Finally, be in class to complete the course evaluation. Write down what you have seen. Do this for negative experiences as well as for positive experiences. Reward your instructors for including diverse topics and encouraging difficult dialogues. These evaluations are read by the department and taken seriously. This is an easy and anonymous way to let the administration know that you value diversity.

Exercise for Dealing with Instructor/Faculty Bias and Discrimination

DIRECTIONS: Please read the scenario and rank order your responses on a scale of 1 to 5, with 5 meaning the most multiculturally responsible and 1 meaning the least multiculturally responsible.

You have been waiting to speak with your instructor for half an hour to review your math homework. You are concerned because you do not understand the most recent lecture and there is a test in two days. An Asian male emerges from the office and you enter. As you sit down, your instructor says, "Wow, those people are usually so good at math." You respond by:

_____ Agreeing that, "Yeah, they usually are."

_____ Questioning the use of the phrase, "Those people?"

_____ Pointing out, "Well, sometimes stereotypes are just stereotypes."

_____ Exclaiming, "Wow, you are a racist!"

_____ Remaining silent.

Pick the response that you feel is the most multiculturally responsible for you. Remember that most of the answers have subtle differences that will be more or less attractive answers based on personal differences. After you have rank ordered them, please break into small groups to discuss why you chose your ranking. In addition, discuss the risks involved with each response. The members of each small group will learn more about becoming multiculturally responsible from listening to others and their preferences. There is no right answer, so please focus on *why* people ranked the responses in the way that they did. After the small-group discussions, one member of each group should report to the class as a whole what was learned in their group.

AWARENESS INTO ACTION: SURPASSING ACADEMIC VARIABLES

As this chapter has demonstrated, students need to be aware that they do not all enter the college classroom with the same assumptions and privileges. Whether a person is a member of the majority group striving to become an MRP or is a member of a racial, ethnic, or cultural minority—or a woman—seeking an equal academic playing field both for themselves and for members of other groups, awareness of classroom variables is an important way to surpass them. Become aware of the variables different people experience in the classroom: different concepts of attendance

> **QUOTATION**
>
> *It is your responsibility to change society if you think of yourself as an educated person.*
>
> JAMES BALDWIN

and punctuality, different notions about classroom participation and interaction with instructors, different experiences with language in the classroom, different experiences regarding being singled out or silenced in the classroom, different experiences with bias in textbooks, and different experiences in dealing with discrimination.

In some cases (attendance/punctuality, and participation/interaction), some students may need to adapt these variables by adjusting to the majority, but other students and instructors should be understanding of the variables and adjust their assumptions about what is "right" and "wrong" accordingly. In other cases (the remaining four variables), all students need to recognize these problems and work to adjust to the classroom situation to move beyond them. Learn how to say, "I am uncomfortable (answering that question, how this is being taught, etc.)." Expressing your personal beliefs can be difficult. If you do not feel comfortable expressing yourself in the moment, then try to speak to your instructor or a trusted advisor after class. Without your feedback, your instructor will not know how to change. Finally, let your instructors know what they are doing right.

CHAPTER AND PERSONAL REVIEW QUESTIONS

1. What are the six classroom variables that students of different races, ethnicities, cultures, and genders may experience?

2. What are some of the variables that students of different races, ethnicities, cultures, and genders may experience regarding punctuality and attendance?

3. What are some of the variables that students of different races, ethnicities, cultures, and genders may experience regarding classroom participation and interaction with the instructor?

4. What are some of the variables that students of different races, ethnicities, cultures, and genders may experience regarding language in the classroom?

5. In what ways are some students singled out and some students silenced in the classroom?

6. In what ways can textbooks sometimes be biased?

7. In what ways can instructors intentionally or unintentionally express bias toward students of different races, ethnicities, cultures, and women?

8. Now that you have learned about the ways racially, ethnically and culturally diverse students, and women experience the academic classroom differently from men and/or those in the majority groups, are you motivated to change your own behaviors and/or call other people on their behaviors to make the classroom a better learning environment for all students? Why or why not? If yes, what steps do you plan to take?

REFERENCE

Loewen, J. W. (1996). *Lies my teacher told me: Everything your American history textbook got wrong*. New York: Simon & Schuster.

CHAPTER 5

Racial, Ethnic, Cultural, and Gender Variables in College Life

BEFORE YOU READ

1. What were your expectations about the out-of-classroom college experience (housing, sports, extracurricular activities) when you first arrived on campus? Has that experience been what you expected or has it been different?

2. What issues or complications do you think might arise between roommates of different races, ethnicities, and/or cultures? Have you experienced any of these?

3. How do you think members of different races, ethnicities, cultures, and genders might experience participation in the Greek system?

4. How do you think members of different races, ethnicities, cultures, and genders might experience participation in college sports?

5. How do you think members of different races, ethnicities, cultures, and genders might experience participation in extracurricular activities such as student government, pre-professional groups, the campus newspaper, the college radio station, film society, and so forth?

6. When you first arrived on campus, did you plan to get involved with any campus identity groups? If so, did your expectations about the group or groups you wanted to join meet your needs? If not, why not?

7. In what ways do you think students who want to participate in LGBT, Arab, or Muslim identity groups might encounter resistance on campus?

8. How would you define the term *multiple identities*? Are you a person who is of multiple racial, ethnic, cultural, and/or gender identities? Whether or not you are, what do you think might be some of the conflicts people of multiple identities might experience on campus?

INTRODUCTION

The classroom is not the only place where students experience college life differently. As with academic life, many students hold a typical view of what college life is like outside of the classroom. Many students automatically think that college offers a standard set of options for housing: For the first year in a residential college (as opposed to a commuter college), they will live in a residence hall with students from the same basic educational and economic background; then typically by their second year they will have the option to either join a fraternity or sorority, stick with residence hall life, or get an apartment nearby the campus. The assumption for housing at community colleges is that traditional-college-age students will live with parents for the first year and get an apartment during their second year. Similarly, the typical view of extracurricular life at all colleges is that most students have the option of participating in sports, joining various student organizations such as student government, the radio station, the debate club, a political organization, a religious organization, the campus newspaper, the literary journal, or an identity group such as the African-American Student Coalition or the Asian-American Alliance. The beneficial aspects of extracurricular activities are that you have the choice to participate or not, you can make new friends, your affiliation with extracurricular activities looks good on your résumé, and you can drop out of such activities without penalty. However, as with academics (and indeed with the "real world"), not all students experience campus housing and extracurricular activities in the same way.

THE VARIABLES OF CAMPUS AND OFF-CAMPUS LIFE

College housing and extracurricular life, like academic life, may reflect the values of the dominant racial, ethnic, cultural, and gender groups and as such may conflict with the values of or exclude women and students from diverse backgrounds. Consider the following benefits as touted by one particular residential college's student guidebook regarding housing and extracurricular programs:

- "Although all students are assigned to residence halls for their first year, sophomore year opens up many options, including the option to join fraternities and sororities, move into specialized housing (such as the literary society house, the food co-op, or the quiet residence hall), or move to an off-campus apartment if so desired."

- "The college offers a wide variety of sports options for students, with a special emphasis on the sports for which this college is well-placed nationally, such as football, lacrosse, and wrestling. Other options may include a variety of men's and women's sports."

- "A wide variety of student organizations exist on campus to enhance students' educational experience via extracurricular activities. Among the many student organizations are the campus newspaper *The Southerner*, our FM classical radio station, several pre-law, pre-med, and pre-government student groups, and special-interest groups such as the literary magazine *Seven Gables* and the American Film Society, which focuses on bringing classic American films to campus."

- "For those students interested in exploring their own racial, ethnic, or cultural backgrounds further and in conjunction with other students from similar backgrounds, the college endorses a variety of student identity groups, such as the Women's Center, the Black and Latin Student Alliance, and the Hillel, a Jewish student organization."

The preceding housing and extracurricular options sound wonderful and enticing, but in reality, how accommodating are these housing and extracurricular options to all students, regardless of race, ethnicity, culture (including sexual orientation and ability status), and gender? In the following sections we will explore the variables of the outside-of-class campus experience in more detail, focusing on housing, sports, extracurricular options, and identity groups.

Out-of-Classroom Variable #1: Housing

The rosy picture the student guidebook in the preceding section paints about housing can certainly be true for some students. In their first year, students may end up with roommate situations that work wonderfully or at least well enough so that there is a minimum of conflict or discomfort. Students may also be able to adapt easily to their options after the first year, pledging to and being accepted by fraternities or sororities, making new friends and opting to live with these friends on or off campus, living alone or with a dating partner, or moving into special-interest campus living situations with a minimum of complications.

However, housing is often complicated by a number of issues related to student diversity. Do not assume that all students have the choice to live on campus, as a large percentage of students at any given school live off campus. Remember, too, that economic disparity prevents some students from being able to attend college in another state or even another city that is not their current home. Many students with limited financial resources may need to commute from home to attend classes and are therefore unable to take advantage of campus living, something that might be considered a privilege. Still other students may need to live at home because they have children, a full-time job, and/or cultural obligations that dictate they must remain close to and in support of their extended families and communities. When you meet new students during your first-year orientation, do not automatically assume that they do or can live on campus. Becoming a multiculturally responsible person (MRP) involves asking people questions before making such assumptions.

CAMPUS HOUSING

When students are able to opt for campus housing, issues related to racial, ethnic, and cultural differences may complicate the living situation. Even seemingly minor incidents can be misinterpreted. For instance, Sharon, a European-American Jewish student, moved into her campus room a few days prior to her roommate, Kathryn, an African-American student. Sharon was looking forward to meeting Kathryn, hoping that they would get along as roommates. As Sharon walked through the door to meet Kathryn for the first time, she found Kathryn pulling out the decorative paper Sharon had put into drawers of the one desk in the room. Kathryn, who had no idea that Sharon had put it there and who was really only removing the paper in an effort to break the ice, said, "Oh hi, the last person who lived here must have put this paper in. It's so WASPy and preppy!" Already hurt that Kathryn had not responded to her friendly gesture to decorate the room before Kathryn moved in, and bothered by the assumption that her personal tastes instantly negated her Jewishness, Sharon further made the assumption that Kathryn's "preppy" comment meant that Kathryn equated "preppy" with White. Sharon never told Kathryn that she was the one who had decorated the desk drawers, so when Sharon acted irritated about it, Kathryn assumed from prior experiences with racism that Sharon's huffiness

> **REFLECTION**
>
> Have you ever assumed that someone did not like you because of your race, ethnicity, or culture and later found out that your assumption was the result of a misunderstanding? Have you ever been accused of being biased when you knew the accusation was a result of a misunderstanding? How did you deal with the situation?

reflected her disappointment in finding out that her roommate was Black, and decided that Sharon was racist. Through lack of communication, the roommates never quite got along after this initial meeting.

Although there are blatant racists, anti-Semites, and other bigoted people in the world, communication among roommates can be improved when roommates can discuss their differences openly. Sharon could have opted to talk openly with Kathryn about the desk paper instead of simply acting irritated and writing her off immediately as anti-White. At the same time, Kathryn could have asked Sharon why she seemed irritated rather than immediately writing her off as a racist. Living with someone of a different culture can be an enriching experience. Students can build friendships by inquiring about the cultural backgrounds of others. For example, a student from Kenya can overcome a racial stereotype about African people being naturally fast runners by explaining to his American roommate that his uncle from Kenya performs well in the Boston Marathon because Kenyans run every day as their major form of transportation. An individual of Mexican-American heritage can deepen her roommate's limited understanding of the richness of Mexican culture by talking about how her grandparents emigrated to America from a small town under the shadow of the ancient Mayan pyramids. Some students may experience negative encounters with culturally diverse roommates, but the value of cross-cultural sharing far outweighs the negatives.

Sexual orientation carries with it its own complex issues when it comes to roommate situations. The majority of individuals make the assumption that people are attracted to and date people of the opposite sex. Therefore, when two people of the same gender are paired together as roommates, there is often an assumption that the roommates are heterosexual. However, when one roommate is suspected of being gay or bisexual or openly reveals his or her interest in the same or both genders, the heterosexual roommate often thinks, "Does my roommate want me? Does my roommate find me attractive?" Most often a lesbian, gay, or bisexual person is not interested in dating his or her roommate. Lesbian, gay, or bisexual individuals are typically interested in respect and acceptance from their roommates. When people are unnecessarily anxious around their roommates because of their sexual orientation or when they assume that their roommates are always "checking them out," they create a rift. Similarly, when lesbian, gay, or bisexual roommates assume that their heterosexual roommates are bigoted, or when they do in fact consciously or unconsciously objectify their roommates, a rift can be created as well.

For instance, Derek identified himself as a gay man to his roommate, Paul, by saying, "By the way, I'm totally into guys." Because they had just met and because Paul did not have any prior experience dealing with lesbian, gay, or bisexual people, Paul did not understand why Derek was sharing his sexual orientation, particularly in such a blunt way, and he immediately thought that Derek was sexually and romantically interested in him. To make

REFLECTION

If you are heterosexual and have lesbian, gay, and/or bisexual friends, how did you respond the first time a friend came out to you? Has your way of responding changed over time? If you are lesbian, gay, or bisexual, how did you approach coming out to your friends for the first time? Has your approach to coming out changed over time?

sure that Derek understood that he was not interested in return, Paul unintentionally insulted Derek by saying, "Well, I do not want you looking at me when I am getting dressed." For his part, Derek was perhaps a little too blunt with Paul about his sexual orientation insofar as he used humor so that he would not sound as if were apologizing to Paul for his sexual orientation, and he also immediately put Paul in the "homophobe" category when Paul responded inappropriately instead of talking it through with Paul further. Paul failed to recognize that Derek was actually trying to create a friendship by being open and humorous about his sexual orientation, and Derek failed to recognize that Paul might not necessarily be homophobic, just relatively new to the topic and a little surprised at the bluntness of Derek's method of coming out.

A more important conversation that Paul and Derek need to have is how they are going to respond when their romantic partners come over to visit. Paul may learn to be more comfortable with Derek's sexuality in an abstract form, but because images of homosexual intimacy are still largely hidden in the media and in other aspects of American life, he may find it awkward to come home after his late class and find two men kissing each other. Derek will be just as socially conditioned as Paul to not blink twice at the thought of coming home to find a man and a woman kissing. However, it would be a double standard for Paul not to abide by the same ground rules as Derek regarding visits from partners. Discussing what the fair ground rules are and mutually abiding by them would create a healthier roommate living situation.

Exercise for Facilitating Roommate Respect and Communication

DIRECTIONS: The examples of Sharon and Kathryn and Derek and Paul illustrate how communication can be tricky between roommates from different racial, ethnic, and cultural groups. From the following list, put a check mark next to the items that you think would help improve roommate communication and respect and put an "x" next to the items that you think would hinder roommate communication and respect.

_____ **1.** Ask your roommate questions about his or her family and neighborhood.

_____ **2.** Demonstrate your support of your roommate's race/ethnicity/culture by attempting to adopt some of his or her racial, ethnic, or cultural slang.

_____ **3.** Let your roommate know that you will try to come to terms with his or her sexuality, but for the time being suggest that you not talk about it while you think about it.

_____ **4.** Draw a line in the sand for yourself concerning what you will and will not discuss with your roommate about race, ethnicity, and/or culture.

_____ **5.** Have a dinner party in your residence hall lounge, to which your roommate brings two guests and you bring two guests.

_____ **6.** Make a point of discussing politics as often as possible so that all political issues, including those related to race/ethnicity/culture, are eventually covered.

_____ **7.** Ask your roommate about his or her hobbies or interests, even if you're not necessarily interested in the same things.

_____ **8.** Invite your friends over every weekend so that your roommate can get to know you better through your friends.

_____ **9.** Suggest to your roommate that you join a campus organization together—not necessarily an identity organization but any organization of mutual interest, such as the radio station.

_____ **10.** Learn when to step back and give your roommate his or her own space.

Some answers might be less obvious that others, but we suggest that items 1, 5, 7, 9, and 10 are good ways to foster respect and communication (without forcing it, which is why 10 is a good thing), while items 2, 3, 4, 6, and 8 are less desirable ways to foster respect and communication; adopting someone else's racial/ethnic/cultural slang might be seen as mimicking and condescending toward your roommate (#2), putting off important conversations for your own peace of mind is not the way to solve issues (#3), being rigid about identity discussions puts roadblocks in the way of reaching understanding (#4), externalizing political issues rather than dealing with them on a personal level deflects real human interaction (#6), and expecting your friends to help forge a relationship with your roommate for you isn't the solution (#8).

OFF-CAMPUS HOUSING, SPECIAL-INTEREST RESIDENCE HALLS, AND FRATERNITY/SORORITY LIVING

Choosing to move from an assigned-roommate on-campus living situation to an off-campus apartment or a special-interest residence hall after the first year most likely will involve living with friends with whom you have already established trust and understanding. As such, there is not much need to discuss such living situations in terms of possible racial, ethnic, and cultural conflicts. In such situations, men and women may need to learn how to live

REFLECTION

Think about the following questions regarding Greek organizations:

1. Imagine a male who has joined a fraternity. What does he look like? What type of person is he?
2. Imagine a female who has joined a sorority. What does she look like? What type of person is she?
3. What is the difference between the North-American Interfraternity Conference, National Panhellenic Conference, National Pan-Hellenic Council, Multicultural Greek Council, and National Association of Latino Fraternal Organizations?

with each other comfortably and respectfully for the first time outside of the family, but the fact that established friendships are already involved ought to smooth the transition. When it comes to single-sex fraternities and sororities, however, there are a number of racial, ethnic, cultural, and gender variables to understand in terms of becoming an MRP.

Many students tend to think of sororities and fraternities as White organizations. In addition, they may not be aware that there are culturally diverse Greek organizations, such as the nine historically Black fraternities and sororities that make up the National Pan-Hellenic Council, local or national associations of Hispanic-American and Asian-American fraternities and sororities often joined together into a Multicultural Greek Council, and a National Association of Latino Fraternal Organizations. Despite the fact that alternatives to White Greek organizations do exist, White Greek organizations and Multicultural Greek organizations often remain racially and ethnically segregated except on rare occasions when a member of another race or ethnicity is admitted. Furthermore, White Greek organizations typically have their own on-campus houses while racially and ethnically diverse fraternities and sororities often do not. This racial and ethnic segregation discourages communication and understanding between groups and sometimes manifests itself in ugly ways, as the following examples illustrate:

- A burning cross was placed on the lawn of the Alpha Kappa Alpha sorority at a large Southern university. Alpha Kappa Alpha was the first Black sorority to move into sorority row. Years later, the problem persisted, with the sororities throwing several theme parties called "Who Rides the Bus?," which featured members in blackface and Afro wigs mocking the Civil Rights Movement.

- During a fraternity initiation ceremony, the fraternity members burned a cross while wearing Civil War uniforms and waving Confederate flags.

- A fraternity held a "Viva Mexico" party for which the invitations were "expired green cards" and there was a "border control" guard at the door.

- Members of a fraternity performed a homecoming skit involving blackface. The university placed the fraternity on probation, ordered the group to hire and pay for a diversity speaker, and mandated that its members participate in a program on the history and implications of blackface.

These incidents cause bad feelings on both sides, and though university officials may step in and directly address the issues involved, the incidents nonetheless reinforce long-standing racial and ethnic barriers. The fraternities and sororities often do not understand that they have done anything wrong, and feel that someone is being "too sensitive" about a lighthearted party. Others feel offended and oppressed, often shocked by the lack of sensitivity and racial/ethnic awareness demonstrated by their peers.

The lack of cross-racial or cross-ethnic communication between White and racially/ethnically diverse fraternities and sororities is a major missed opportunity for promoting interracial/interethnic interaction among college students. The college community where many different groups inhabit the same space is fertile ground for preparing future leaders to live in a multicultural world. There are cases where historically White fraternities and sororities and racially/ethnically diverse fraternities and sororities have worked together, such as through intramural athletics and charitable events, and there are some emerging new trends in which sororities and fraternities that have houses (as mentioned, typically White Greek organizations) offer to host and co-sponsor events with Greek organizations that do not have houses. Unfortunately, these types of collaboration do not receive the same publicity as negative interactions. Hopefully, such activities and initiatives to promote communication and interaction among Greek organizations on campus will continue to proliferate, and negative incidents like those mentioned in this section will become increasingly rare.

In addition to racial and ethnic disparities within the Greek system, gender disparities also exist within the system more often than not. Sometimes these disparities can be linked to an overall lesser interest in the Greek system among women than among men. For instance, at many smaller liberal arts colleges, sororities and fraternities are viewed as elitist organizations by both men and women, with women viewing Greek organizations as historically male, sexist organizations. Many such colleges have banned Greek organizations from campus altogether. However, the banning of Greek organizations from college and university campuses is the exception rather than the rule, with many colleges and universities continuing to offer fraternity and sorority living as an option, if a limited one for women. More often than not, women have less of an opportunity

> ## REFLECTION
>
> How many fraternities are there on your campus? How many sororities are there? Of the existing fraternities and sororities, which gender has the better housing?

> ## REFLECTION
>
> Imagine you are a lesbian, gay, or bisexual student in the Greek system. What would make you want to join a fraternity or sorority? Would you want to come out as a lesbian, gay, or bisexual person to your fraternity or sorority brothers or sisters or would you remain closeted? What might be the consequences if you came out to your brothers and sisters?

to join sororities than men have of joining fraternities simply because there is less sorority housing available. In addition, whether or not they participate in the Greek system, women continue to be exploited by it, with incidents of date rape at fraternities still outnumbering such incidents elsewhere on campus and still persisting as a major problem nationwide.

One overlooked area in the Greek system is sexual orientation. The assumption most students make within single-sex fraternities and sororities is that their members are heterosexual. However, this is not always the case. Such assumptions exclude lesbian, gay, and bisexual students from the advantages (peer group bonding, often better housing than that found in residence halls, etc.) of fraternity and sorority living. Should they pledge and be accepted in a fraternity or sorority, lesbian, gay, and bisexual students are likely to experience a bonding system that—because it involves bonding between individuals of the same gender—denies homosexuality in often emphatically homophobic ways (e.g., humiliating pledges during the initiation process by calling them "queer" or the like). Because of fear, many lesbian, gay, or bisexual students either avoid the Greek system altogether (which restricts their freedom in terms of housing options) or remain closeted within the system.

There are some success stories in which some fraternities and sororities are accepting and supportive of their lesbian, gay, or bisexual members, and indeed there are a few chapters of some fraternities and sororities that predominantly consist of lesbian, gay, or bisexual members, but more often than not homosexuality is openly discouraged in the Greek system. As such, many colleges are using the Lambda 10 (or L10) Project, which has created guidelines for fraternities and sororities to help create what they term Greek Safe Zone Ally programs. Individuals involved in these programs agree to listen openly, confront homophobic jokes or comments, keep information confidential, and educate themselves regarding LGBT concerns. These programs expect that people will have differing views on LGBT issues and that some people may not agree with same-sex relationships at all. As such, the focus of being an ally is to be emotionally supportive of LGBT people as people and to treat them with respect.

Exercise for Facilitating Diversity Within and Across the Greek System

Remember that fraternities and sororities are private organizations in which students of similar interests and worldviews pledge and are accepted for the very reason that they would be like-minded and get along easily with their brothers and sisters within those organizations. So, we want to be careful not to advocate that Greek organizations should go co-ed, or that Black or Hispanic fraternities and sororities start pledging White students. However, the exclusivity of fraternities and sororities is problematic in that exclusivity often exists at the expense of diversity. Keeping both sides of the coin in mind, there are nonetheless many ways that fraternities and sororities can (and sometimes do) do a better job of contributing to an overall atmosphere of respect for gender and racial/ethnic/cultural diversity on campus.

On the following list, put a check mark next to each item that you feel fraternities/sororities could do to facilitate respect for diversity and/or gender, and put an "x" next to each item that is misguided in terms of respecting women and diverse groups.

_____ **1.** Co-sponsor parties with other fraternities and/or sororities on campus or with student identity groups.

_____ **2.** Eliminate homophobic and/or sexist bonding practices during initiation, such as forcing pledges to wear dresses, using homophobic language, and making pledges provide proof of sexual conquests.

_____ **3.** Pledge one person per year who is a member of a different race, ethnicity, or culture than the majority of the fraternity or sorority members.

_____ **4.** Ask members of the fraternity or sorority to avoid public displays of racism, classism, sexism, and homophobia.

_____ **5.** If no multicultural Greek organizations exist on campus, work with the administration and interested students toward bringing chapters of such organizations to campus.

_____ **6.** Give money to a soup kitchen or AIDS organization to demonstrate to the college student body and administration that the fraternity or sorority has made a contribution to charity.

_____ **7.** Create or modify organizational guidelines to incorporate measures to deal swiftly and judiciously with incidents of racism, sexism, homophobia, ethnocentrism, and so forth among fraternity or sorority members.

_____ **8.** Hire as the house parent, chef, or caretaker someone from a racial, ethnic, or cultural group different from most of the members of the fraternity or sorority, as a means of speaking to diversity.

_____ **9.** Host or support events within the house or elsewhere on campus focused on diversity.

_____ **10.** Create a house diversity sheet that highlights the diversity that already exists within the fraternity or sorority and demonstrates that not all members are of the exact same backgrounds.

As with the roommate exercise earlier in this chapter, some answers here are less obvious than others, but our feeling is that items 1, 2, 5, 7, and 9 are the most productive things fraternities and sororities could do to demonstrate a true (and active) respect for diversity on campus. The other items on the list are misguided because they are about tokenism rather than about a real commitment to diversity (items 3 and 8), they are about hiding problems related to diversity rather than solving them (item 4), or they are about paying lip service to diversity rather than being truly invested in fostering it (items 6 and 10). Although giving money to a charity (item 6) is certainly a good thing, it should not be the only thing the Greek organization ever does to make a contribution.

Out-of-Classroom Variable #2: Sports

Surely we do not need to think about diversity issues in college sports, right? Sports are simply about the game: practice, winning and losing, and team building, not racism, sexism, and heterosexism, right? Of course sports are about camaraderie, doing one's personal best, and other positive things. But sports can give a person seeking to become an MRP as much of a workout as can any other area of college life. Consider the following incidents from college sports:

> **REFLECTION**
>
> Have you seen any recent sport films, such as *Remember the Titans, A League of Their Own, Bend It Like Beckham, Glory Road,* or *Coach Carter*? If so, how did these films present themes related to racial/ethnic/cultural/gender differences? How did these themes mirror your own experience with sports and diversity?

- In 2006, Penn State women's basketball coach Rene Portland was given a slap on the wrist by university administrators and warned to cease discriminating against athletes she perceived to be lesbian. This was in response to the allegations of Jennifer Harris, a player who said she was dismissed from the team for being a lesbian. Portland's feelings on the subject have been documented back to the mid-1980s, when she told the *Chicago Sun-Times* that she did not want lesbians on her team.

- Paul Hornung, a sports commentator for Notre Dame football and a football Hall of Fame inductee, indicated that Notre Dame should lower its academic standards to attract better Black football players, thus perpetuating the stereotype of African-American football players as less intelligent than White football players.

- A former place-kicker for University of Colorado football, Katie Hnida, revealed to *Sports Illustrated* in 2004 that she had suffered years of verbal and physical abuse from her male teammates. She had been called sexually graphic names, groped during huddles, and allegedly raped by a teammate. Rather than come to her defense, her coach merely referred to her place on the team as a "distraction."

As these examples illustrate, incidents of racial, ethnic, cultural, and gender bias exist up and down the spectrum of college sports, just as they exist in all facets of college life and in all facets of life outside of college. College is a microcosm of American society as a whole, and so unfortunately it mirrors the same problems that occur elsewhere. It is the duty of every multiculturally responsible individual to stand up against any act that labels people negatively and violates their rights.

RACIAL AND ETHNIC BIAS IN COLLEGE SPORTS

The first two incidents of bias in college sports from the preceding bulleted list demonstrate that racial and ethnic bias are not simply things of the past, despite great strides made by African Americans, Hispanic Americans, Jews, and others in the athletic arena. For instance, consider how both college and professional sports teams have been criticized and scrutinized for using Native Americans as team mascots. A number of professional teams use Native-American mascots, including the Chiefs, the Braves, the Indians, and the Redskins. The same is true of college teams, many of whom argue that Native-American mascots are complimentary. They are used as a way of demonstrating the team's bravery and strength. Yet, Native-American organizations have been working to remove such mascots from sports teams since the 1960s, arguing that such images as the "red-faced, hook-nosed, grinning buffoon" representing the Cleveland Indians, "does not resemble any indigenous peoples. The name and logo do not 'honor' Native peoples, but perpetuate racist stereotypes" (Shaw, 2003). Further, because the images of Native American chiefs are sacred symbols among tribes, having a person parade around in a headdress at a sporting event is like having a person dressed up like the Pope at halftime. Surely having a Pope mascot would offend Catholics, Native-American spokespersons state, as a stereotypical Rabbi as a team mascot would offend Jews.

Recently, the NCAA has prohibited colleges or universities with hostile or abusive mascots from hosting any NCAA championship competitions. In addition, in the last 25 years, over a dozen schools have changed either their team mascots or team nicknames. Other schools have refused to schedule athletic competitions with schools that use Native-American nicknames or mascots. One reason schools might take such a strong stance about athletic teams with which they compete is to be respectful of their Native-American student body. School spirit often involves creating posters or large papier-mâché mascots that involve aggressive acts. Therefore, it would not be uncommon to find banners that read "Lions claw the Indians," "Lions eat the Indians," and "Indians will be destroyed!" Imagine what it might be like to be a Native-American student on campus with this type of "school spirit."

Resisting dehumanizing sports mascots parallels the rejection of the Confederate flag (a symbol that for many represented the embracement of slavery), which was for many years raised during college sporting events in the South. Although the Confederate flag is no longer considered an acceptable symbol in sports, college or otherwise, other forms of racial and ethnic bias—beyond the symbolic—continue to exist. For one thing, while the presence of African-American and other minority athletes has grown considerable in college sports over the last 50 years, there remain relatively few minority coaches, which mirrors the primarily White-controlled professional sports industry in which African-American athletes are faced with few coaching options once their athletic careers are over. The good news is that systematic attempts (broader searches, more representative search committees, stakeholders meetings) are being made to hire more coaches and administrators that reflect the diversity of the players in major sports such as professional football and basketball.

Another major roadblock for minority students in college is that, while few would argue that minority students are denied access to college sports, many make the assumption that participation in sports is the primary reason minority students (typically African-American students) attend college in the first place. For example, Michael, a White student, was introduced to Tim, a friend of a friend, and an African-American student, for the first time. Within moments after meeting Tim, Michael asked Tim about his prospects for making the college's basketball team, what position he played, and what city he was from. Tim did not respond verbally, but his facial expressions were those of an individual who was first baffled and then insulted. Why did Tim register these expressions? Because he had absolutely no interest in basketball, was in fact not particularly athletic, grew up in an affluent suburb of Boston, and had been accepted to the college early admission because of his excellent high school grades and high SAT scores. Tim was deeply offended that Michael automatically assumed he was an athlete from "the hood" and probably got into the college on a basketball scholarship.

Exercise for Dealing with Racial and Ethnic Bias in Sports

Given the preceding scenario, which of the following questions could Michael have asked that would have been more multiculturally responsible? Please rank order your responses from 1 to 5, with 5 meaning the most multiculturally responsible and 1 meaning the least multiculturally responsible.

_____ "Hi Tim. I'm a major sports fan. Do you participate in sports?"

_____ "Hi Tim. You look like a real ringer, do you shoot hoops?"

_____ "Hi Tim. You wouldn't happen to be a ball player would you?"

_____ "Hi Tim. We could really use a guy with your height on the basket-ball team. Do you have time to play?"

_____ "Hi Tim. What type of things do you do for fun?"

After you have rank ordered the responses, please break into small groups to discuss why you ranked each question in the way you did. You will learn more about becoming multiculturally responsible by listening to others and their preferences. There is no right answer, so please focus on why people chose the particular responses they chose. Remember that most of the answers involve subtle differences. In addition, discuss the risks involved with each response. After the small-group discussion, one member of each group should report what his or her group learned in the small group discussion.

Ethnic bias can also be an issue in college sports, particularly when one considers how frequently Christian beliefs are brought into sports at the expense of those students who are of other religious beliefs, such as Jewish, Muslim, Hindi, or Buddhist students, or those who are agnostic or atheist. At many colleges, it is acceptable for coaches (most of whom, as discussed earlier, are from White, Christian backgrounds) to speak about Christian beliefs during practices, lead their teams in Christian prayers (such as The Lord's Prayer), or even occasionally quote Bible passages in the team's printed itinerary. Students may feel that their religious beliefs are not being respected in such cases, but often will not speak out due to fear of losing the respect of the coach and/or teammates.

GENDER AND SEXUAL ORIENTATION BIAS IN COLLEGE SPORTS

Despite the fact that women have made great strides in the sports world, to the point where such athletes as Jackie Joyner-Kersee, Martina Navratilova, Chris Evert, Mia Hamm, Billie Jean King, Kristi Yamaguchi, Julie Krone, Picabo Street, Sheryl Swoopes, and Mary Lou Retton are as celebrated as their male counterparts, women still face an uphill battle in the sports arena. This is true in both the professional sports world, which is still very much a male-dominated profession, and in college, where women experience a number of barriers to full acceptance as athletes.

First, public comments about women's supposed inability to participate in sports can affect the respect that female athletes receive, with comments about women's biological "limitations" and physical incompatibility with sports still quite common. Other stereotypes are that women are too emotional to play sports, women may become pregnant and leave sports, and that it is against women's nature to be passionate about a competitive game.

Second, female athletes are not as respected as they should be, because—despite the world famous names listed in the preceding paragraph—there remains a dearth of positive examples of famous female athletes who have been celebrated in the media to the degree of their male counterparts, despite the existence of many clearly deserving women. For instance, many people would not be able to name the greatest female athlete of the first half of the twentieth century—one of the pioneers for acceptance of women in athletics—Babe Didrikson Zaharias. Didrikson Zaharias first excelled as an All-America high school basketball player. In the 1932 Summer Olympics, she won gold medals and broke her own world records in both javelin and 80-meter hurdles. In addition, she was awarded the silver medal for high jumping (she cleared a world-record height, but was ruled ineligible for the gold because her jump technique—clearing the bar headfirst—was considered unorthodox at the time). She began her second Hall of Fame career on the amateur golf tour in 1934, and went on to 35 career victories, including three U.S. Opens and an unprecedented 17 consecutive tournament titles from 1946 to 1947. She was one of the founding members of the Ladies Professional Golf Association (LPGA) in 1950. Given all of her accomplishments, it is surprising that she is not as well known as such great male athletes of the first half of the century as Jesse Owens, Babe Ruth, Sugar Ray Robinson, and Lou Gehrig.

> **REFLECTION**
>
> Women in the past 30 years have attained increased prominence in sports. Most people, even those who do not follow sports, can probably name at least 20 famous female athletes. But how many women athletes from the first half of the twentieth century can you name? Why do you think that is?

Another reason women athletes have difficulty finding acceptance as athletes is that sports events require money, and most of that money, in both the professional world and in college, is still in the hands of men. This is particularly true with team sports that are still considered primarily the domain of men. In recent years, women have excelled in team sports such as soccer and basketball, and popularity is on the rise in these sports. But the stereotype still persists that women are better at sports such as tennis and golf, and men are better at sports such as football and basketball. Inevitably,

> **REFLECTION**
>
> How often do you see or read about women's sporting events on television and in the newspaper compared to men's sporting events? Of the women's sporting events that are covered, how many are team-oriented sports rather than individual sports like golf, tennis, and gymnastics? Why do you think this is the case?

these stereotypes affect the money machine, the result being that most colleges and universities do not offer as many options to female athletes across the board (but particularly with regard to women's team sports) as they offer to men. In most cases, women's athletics are under-funded compared to men's athletics.

When it comes to sexual orientation, the world of sports is famously homophobic, both for women and for men. Increasingly, lesbians in the sports world have gained prominence, with such world-class athletes as Martina Navratilova, Billie Jean King, and Sheryl Swoopes publicly coming out of the closet. However, resistance is strong. One recent example, as cited previously, involved Jennifer Harris, a basketball player at Penn State, who claimed she was kicked off of the basketball team by her coach because of her perceived sexual orientation. In another case, at the University of Florida, Andrea Zimbardi claimed that she was suspended and later released from the softball team because of her perceived sexual orientation. The student was able to cite, with evidence, several incidents when her softball coach and assistant coach made inappropriate remarks about lesbian women. Two other former players, who had also been suspended from the team, cited similar experiences. Such incidents are becoming more and more common as lesbian athletes gain prominence nationwide, and indeed worldwide.

For gay male athletes, the situation is different but no less troublesome. While lesbian athletes are coming out of the closet in greater and greater numbers, gay or bisexual male athletes are still largely remaining in the closet, due to intense homophobia in male sports. The common stereotype of women athletes is that, because they choose to participate

> **REFLECTION**
>
> How many openly lesbian, gay, or bisexual athletes can you name? Of those, how many are women and how many are men? Why do you think there are not more openly gay male football, basketball, baseball, or hockey players: Because they do not exist or because they are not allowed to be open? In addition, how many transgender athletes can you name? How will the issue of sexual reassignment surgery affect competitive sports?

in a supposedly "male" activity like sports, many of them are lesbian. Conversely, the stereotype that gay and bisexual men are more interested in supposedly "female" activities such as arts, design, and fashion means that they are viewed as incompatible with sports. Although some stereotypes have a basis in reality, the notion that gay and bisexual men are not interested in sports is sharply contradicted by the many nonprofessional gay sports teams in existence and the popularity of gay sporting events such as the Gay Games. As a result of stereotypes and homophobia, however, very few male athletes at either the professional or college level have publicly come out of the closet. Those who have, such as Greg Louganis, a four-time Olympic gold-medal-winning diver, have perhaps been able to come out because the sports in which they participate are less prone to homophobia than team sports like football or baseball. Gay and bisexual men in team sports may remain closeted until they have retired, such as Esera Tuaolo, a former NFL football player.

Exercise for Counteracting Sports Stereotypes

In America and in many other countries, the popular stereotype is that heterosexual women and gay men are not interested in or adept at sports, while heterosexual men and lesbian women are interested in and adept at sports. An exception to these stereotypes, but a stereotype in itself, is that African-American women (indeed all African Americans) are naturally athletic. If one speaks in generalities and crunches numbers, perhaps there is some truth to the stereotypes, insofar as there are more well-known male athletes than female athletes, there are significantly more out-of-the-closet lesbian athletes than there are out-of-the-closet gay male athletes, and both African-American male and female athletes have excelled in the world of sports overall more than any other racial/ethnic/cultural minority group. However, throughout this book we have emphasized that generalizations are impediments to multiculturally responsible development. Train yourself to "think outside of the box" by doing some Internet research. Locate websites and/or articles related to the following:

_____ **1.** Women's professional and college athletic organizations

_____ **2.** Gay men's athletic organizations and events

_____ **3.** Men's knitting or quilting organizations

_____ **4.** Women's boxing associations

_____ **5.** African-American female poets, philosophers, and artists

_____ **6.** African American male poets, philosophers, and artists

_____ **7.** Lesbian poets, philosophers, and artists

None of the above will prove that people who go against the stereotype can not also simultaneously go with the stereotype (e.g., gay men who are into sports may also be into art/culture, and African-American women poets can also be into sports). However, this exercise is designed to expand upon those stereotypes and encourage thinking outside the box.

Out-of-Classroom Variable #3: Extracurricular Activities

For those students who are interested in business, law, or government, most colleges and universities offer pre-professional organizations, which students can join to get a head start on their careers or simply to practice skills that will help them get ahead in the "real world." Additionally, most campuses feature a variety of other extracurricular organizations that might also be considered pre-professional. For instance, those interested in getting into radio and television might become involved with the college radio station or TV station (if the college funds these programs); those interested in going into publishing or journalism might get involved with a variety of campus publications such as the college newspaper, literary journal, or other publication; and those interested in a career in the arts might sign themselves up to be a part of the college theater group, film society, or art appre-

> **REFLECTION**
>
> What types of pre-professional extracurricular groups exist at your college or university? How might some of these organizations be under-representative of diversity? How might the situation be improved?

ciation society. All of these organizations provide excellent opportunities for students to learn, grow, and get a head start in their future careers. As with all facets of campus life, though perhaps to a lesser extent in this arena than in housing and sports, extracurricular activities may involve variables in which not all students feel they have the same opportunities as other students from majority groups.

Because student government represents the entirety of the student body and most closely reflects the full array of concerns students will face in the outside world, it is in some ways the most important of student extracurricular organizations in college. Ideally, student government should reflect the diversity of the student body, as American government should reflect the diversity of American society. However, as in American society, some campuses involve such diversity that the student government cabinet is not large enough to have someone represent each aspect of diversity. On the other side of the coin, some campuses may not be as diverse as they could be, resulting in a student government that represents the voices of only the dominant racial, ethnic, and cultural groups, and there may continue to be an uneven representation of women in student government. In either case, student government organizations should strive to be as representative and diverse as they can be.

Student government can employ several strategies to better represent the student body. First, members of student government can appoint individuals to cabinet positions who are currently involved in other organizations. An individual who is active in multiple groups will possess a deeper awareness of the overall needs of students than a student who is strictly interested in student government itself. Second, the student government needs to communicate effectively with other student groups. This may involve inviting liaisons from each student group to attend student government meetings. Finally, each member of student government should be an MRP. Student leaders should be aware of their own diversity, be aware of the diversity on their campus, and be able to effectively communicate about diversity issues. As the most visible leaders on campus, students involved in government have the ability to make important changes on campus.

Exercise for Assessing Your Place in Student Government

Please take a moment and answer the following questions:

1. Do you believe that student government represents your interests (e.g., they plan a budget that financially supports activities in which you are interested and they advocate for issues in which you are invested)?

2. What are the demographics of your college student president and vice president? If you do not know, please stop answering these questions and take a moment to find out.

3. What types of people (e.g., race, ethnicity, culture, personality, hobbies) do you think are involved in student government at your college?

4. Why would you be interested in joining student government?

5. Why would you not be interested in joining student government?

6. Do you think you can make a difference by joining student government?

Take a minute to examine your answers. Were you not interested in joining because of other time commitments or because you felt unsure about the job duties? Did you feel that you would not belong or "fit into" student government?

There is a place for all students regardless of their race, ethnicity, culture, gender, socioeconomic status, ability status, sexual orientation, personality, or perspective in student government, just as long as students who want to get involved have the drive to represent the entire student body. Diversity in student government adds strength to the organization.

Student government organizations can accomplish a great deal on campus. For instance, student government can have a major influence on how funds are distributed among student groups on campus. It can step in when students feel that the college administration has not responded satisfactorily to incidents of campus discrimination. It can get students who are not involved in student government motivated to care about and participate in campus affairs in other ways. In short, it can have a strong effect on the overall climate of the campus.

> **REFLECTION**
>
> What students are involved in student government at your college or university? Are any groups not represented in student government? Why do you think this occurs? What could be done to add more diversity to student government on your campus?

Beyond student government, other pre-professional extracurricular groups on campus may not reflect diversity as well as they could, so it is the job of the MRP to get involved in making changes so that the college or university experience is one that benefits everyone on campus. For instance, if the campus newspaper has a politically slanted bias, it is the job of the MRP to make sure that voices of all students on campus are represented in the newspaper, even if those voices might not match the MRP's own political views (of course, there are limits in either direction and no one needs to hear the voice of a hate-filled fanatic). At the campus radio or television station, it is the responsibility of the MRP to ensure that all students share in and benefit from the programming of the station (e.g., a radio station should offer a variety of musical and public interest options, not just one style of musical programming or one group's public interest programming). Pre-law and pre-business groups should not be politically slanted to the point where the voices of diverse students are shut out, thereby shutting out those students' future options in these professions. Finally, literature, music, and arts groups may strive to represent diversity not only within the organizations but also in what they present to the rest of the campus (e.g., an effective literary magazine will not simply publish short stories, poems, and plays by students from one group but by students from all backgrounds and perspectives; an effective guest speakers council could strive to invite speakers to campus who represent a diversity of perspectives and topics; and an effective film society should strive to show not just classic American films primarily written, produced, and directed by White individuals, but also films that mirror the whole spectrum of experiences).

Out-of-Classroom Variable #4: Identity Groups

For those students who feel they are under-represented in or are treated unfairly within other arenas of college life such as academics, housing, sports, and extracurricular activities, or for those students who simply want to explore their own racial, ethnic, cultural, or gender backgrounds more fully with like-minded students, identity groups on campus can be a home away from home. Most colleges sponsor a variety of larger identity groups, such as African American Student Alliance, Women's Coalition, or an Asian Student Union. Depending on the size and diversity of the campus, these larger groups may also involve suborganizations. For instance, an Asian Student Union may have suborganizations for Japanese, Chinese, Thai, Malaysian, Indonesian, Vietnamese, Korean, Taiwanese, and other Asian students. It is the job of the main organization to foster intergroup cooperation and collaboration within these groups and with other student organizations.

Most student identity groups are funded and supported by campus administration or student government. However, it is important to remember that some students either are members of groups that have a harder time getting funding and recognition than other groups (LGBT groups, Muslim and Arab groups, as will be discussed in a following section), and that some students may find that they cross over into multiple groups and therefore "fall through the cracks" of existing identity groups (students who have multiple identities, as will be discussed in a following section). Whether or not they are members of these groups, it is the responsibility of all MRPs to support the right of certain groups to exist and to help facilitate for the needs of those students who "fall through the cracks" to ensure that all students on campus have equal opportunities to join student identity groups reflective of their needs.

LESBIAN, GAY, BISEXUAL, AND TRANSGENDER IDENTITY GROUPS

Lesbian, gay, bisexual, and transgender groups still face an uphill battle in gaining the support of campus administrators on campuses nationwide. This may be due partially to the unpreparedness and/or unwillingness of many students to come out of the closet, resulting in there not being enough "out" students to ask for organizational funding in the first place. But the more likely reason such groups do not exist on many college campuses is because LGBT individuals remain one of the most disenfranchised groups in America today, still not afforded the same civil rights that most other groups have likewise fought to earn over the course of time. For instance, in most states, LGBT individuals can be fired from their jobs or denied housing simply for being gay, and in very few states do LGBT individuals have inheritance or hospital visitation rights should their life partners die or fall ill. Such realities of American society naturally carry through to college campuses, which are, after all, microcosms of the larger society. Legally, campus administrators in many states are not required to recognize LGBT individuals as legitimate minorities. Therefore, typically on more conservative campuses, LGBT organizations are prohibited the right to exist and students often have no legal recourse to discrimination. On some campuses where LGBT groups are recognized and funded, funding may be considerably less than that afforded to other identity groups.

REFLECTION

Is there an LGBT student organization on your campus? If so, how visible is it? How well funded is it (e.g., does it often sponsor events such as guest speakers, films, cultural events, or social gatherings)? If not, why do you think that is the case? Would you be willing to help in some capacity with such an organization? If you did help, would you be concerned that you would be labeled as gay?

ARAB AND MUSLIM IDENTITY GROUPS SINCE 9/11

Student life on college and university campuses does not operate in a vacuum. The same issues that affect people in the larger American society affect everyone on campus, from students, to professors, to staff, to administrators. After the terrorist attacks on September 11, 2001, colleges and universities experienced an upheaval. In fact, colleges may have experienced more culture clash moments related to 9/11 than business, industry, or local government did, because college and university campuses have a way of magnifying and intensifying political hot-button issues due to their smaller comparative size, their insularity, their focus on confronting issues, and their concentrated, diverse populations. Difficulties arose on many college and university campuses when, shortly after 9/11, Muslim and Arab groups (note that these two identities are not synonymous) began to educate people about their religion and culture in response to the sudden backlash they experienced from being equated with the 9/11 terrorists. Their efforts were met with both strong support and hatred. Although the worst of the anti-Arab and Muslim backlash seems to be over, problems persist. After all, war in the Middle East continues, and—as in any wartime situation—suspicion of anyone resembling "the enemy" (no matter how knee-jerk or unfounded that suspicion may be) continues as well. For this reason, those from Arab and/or Muslim backgrounds have often experienced problems gaining funding or acceptance as identity groups on many college campuses.

Knowledge and awareness through education are one way to learn about Arab and Muslim culture and get past negative, stereo-

---

DEFINITION

Arab Americans and *Muslims.* **Arab Americans** are people who come from Algeria, Egypt, Iraq, Jordan, Kuwait, Lebanon, Libya, Palestine, Mauritania, Morocco, Qatar, Saudi Arabia, Yemen, Sudan, Syria, Tunisia, and the United Arab Emirates (Kivel, 2002), a group of countries within a region once known in the West as Arabia and sharing the same basic language (with many dialects), Arabic. People from Iran and Turkey are not considered Arab (their countries are not Arabic-speaking). **Muslims** are persons who follow the faith of Islam. The majority of Arab Americans are Christians, not Muslims. Furthermore, of the one million Muslims in the world, the majority live in non-Arab countries such as Kenya, China, India, and the Philippines (Kivel, 2002).

REFLECTION

Are Arab-American and/or Muslim-American students represented at your college or university? If so, are there Arab and/or Muslim student identity groups in existence? What has the reception been to these groups?

---

typical perceptions. The Western view of Islam, the religion practiced by Muslims, has its roots in the Crusades that began in the eleventh century, in which Christians attempted to forcefully spread Christianity to the Arab world, a byproduct of which was the Western demonization of Muslims as evil people. Hundreds of years later, the stereotypes of Muslims (and by extension Arab Americans) as evil persists in movies and other media, a stereotype reinforced by the cruel and fanatical actions of a terrorist organization that had nothing to do with the beliefs of most Muslims or Arabs, in the Middle East or on American soil. To judge an entire religion and/or region of the world based on a small minority of people is illogical and biased thinking.

MULTIPLE IDENTITIES AND IDENTITY GROUPS

The issue of perceived incompatibility across racial, ethnic, and cultural lines is most noticed by multiple-identity individuals, both inside and outside of college. Do Hispanic women join the college Women's Center or

> ### DEFINITION
>
> **Multiple identities.** While *biracial* or *multiracial* refer to a combination of racial heritages, the term **multiple identities** refers to a combination of identities such as race, ethnicity, sexual orientation, gender, and disability.

the Hispanic Student Assembly? Does a Catholic gay man join the Catholic Student Union or the LGBT Alliance? How does a biracial student who is both Asian and African American fit comfortably within either the African American Student Coalition or the Asian American League? How do students cope with multiple identities, which may appear discrepant from one another?

As we saw in Chapter 2, racial and ethnic identity development proceeds through a number of different stages, identified as pre-encounter/conformity, encounter/dissonance, immersion/emersion, internalization, and integrative awareness. Meanwhile, White people go through their own distinct stages of development: contact, disintegration, reintegration, pseudo-independence, immersion/emersion, and autonomy. Further, LGBT individuals go through

> ### DEFINITION
>
> ### Poston's Bicultural Development Model: Stages of Development Persons from Multiple Cultures May Experience
>
> **Stage 1: Personal Identity:** Individuals are at a young age when personal development factors are often learned from the family.
> **Stage 2: Choice of Group Categorization:** Individuals are pushed to choose an identity in one group.
> **Stage 3: Enmeshment/Denial:** Individuals feel confusion or guilt about having to choose one identity over the other.
> **Stage 4: Appreciation:** Individuals appreciate their multiple identities and start learning about their multiple cultures from an in-depth perspective.
> **Stage 5: Integration:** Individuals become more secure in their multiple identification.

a number of stages themselves: confusion, comparison, tolerance, acceptance, pride, and synthesis; and persons with disabilities go through identity development stages that parallel the racial/ethnic identity stages. So where does this place individuals who cross over into multiple groups, such an individual who has one White parent and one Black parent, or a person who is gay, Jewish, and disabled? Poston (1990) has developed a **Bicultural Development Model** to speak to this question.

Consider the case of Caiti, a 19-year-old college athlete who identifies herself as biracial. Her mother is Peruvian and her father is Haitian. Caiti, a softball player for her college, spent her freshman year adjusting to college life by attending classes and long hours of practice for the softball season. One day at the beginning of her sophomore year, she stopped to think about her life in general and what it meant to be biracial on a college campus. The following are some of the thoughts she pondered:

> Whether I like it or not, people judge me based on my outer appearance. People ask questions such as, "What is your racial/ethnic make-up? Are your parents African American, Hispanic, or White? What are you?" What should I tell them? My father is not really African American, but Haitian American. My mother is from Peru, and identifies with that, rather than as Hispanic. My father died when I was young, and I do not know much about his cultural background. My stepfather is White and I grew up in a neighborhood of mostly White people, so I know little of the cultural heritages of either of my biological parents. When I look at various groups on campus, I have no idea to which I belong. If I chose a Black organization, I'd stand out like a sore thumb because my complexion is so light. If I chose a Hispanic organization, I'd be embarrassed that I do not speak Spanish. Do Hispanic organizations even care if I speak Spanish? I am too ashamed to even find out. If I hang out with mostly White people, which I am most comfortable with since I grew up in a mostly White neighborhood, I am still uncomfortable because I appear different from 100% European-American people. I am one among many, but I do not know my place. Which group should I join? What will people think of me if I choose one group over the other? I am ready to learn and grow, but in which direction, I do not know.

Many college students today face the same dilemma that Caiti faces. In fact, they may identify with more than two groups, not knowing where they belong or being caught between multiple races, ethnicities, and/or cultures. Rebecca Walker, the biracial and bi-ethnic daughter of famed novelist Alice Walker and author of the bestseller *Black, White and Jewish: Autobiography of a Shifting Self*, speaks about her life experiences much like Caiti did.

These issues can be very complicated for students who join identity groups to explore their identities, make friends with people from a similar background, and just "fit in." Sometimes they find that the very groups they joined to feel like they "fit in" make them feel just the opposite. For instance, a lesbian African-American student might experience barriers to acceptance of her lesbianism among her peers in an African-American student group in which many of the members hold religiously conservative views about homosexuality, and at the same time she may experience barriers to acceptance of her Blackness among the predominantly White students in an LGBT student group.

In addition to not "fitting in," students of multiple identities may experience a minimization of their multiple identities. For instance, a student's experience may parallel that of Tiger Woods, who has described himself as *Cablinasian*, a word he coined by stringing together the first syllables of his multiple identity groups: Caucasian-Black-Indian-Asian. Despite his creative attempts to break out of racial categories, however, others did not see it his way. Colin Powell, former Secretary of State, responded to Woods by saying,

"In America, which I love from the depths of my heart and soul, when you look like me, you're black," meaning that despite Woods's multiple identities, most people would label him as Black. Similarly, although most people are familiar with Martin Luther King, Jr., fewer people are aware of his friend Bayard Rustin, who was an openly gay African-American social activist and advisor to King during the Civil Rights movement and was silenced, threatened, and fired from his leadership positions because of his gay identity. He was seen as a liability because of his sexual orientation, but continued behind the scenes and eventually organized the 1963 march on Washington which included King's "I Have a Dream" speech. Because of his multiple identities and public racism and homophobia, he was put into a position where he was forced to minimize one part of his identity at the expense of another.

There is a variety of ways such problems can be addressed by MRPs (whether the MRPs have multiple identities themselves or not). First, MRPs should be aware of and internalize the following Bill of Rights developed by Root (1992). Although Root has conceived the bill of rights in racial terms, it may be applied to all individuals with multiple racial, ethnic, and/or cultural identities:

- Multiracial (ethnic, cultural) individuals have the right to self-definition.
- Multicultural (ethnic, cultural) individuals have the right to self-definition without justifying or defending to others the cultural classification (description or group) that they find personally meaningful.
- Multiracial (ethnic, cultural) individuals must resist the oppressiveness of choosing only one identity group.
- Multiracial (ethnic, cultural) individuals have the right to be complex, ambiguous, and to change their identity over time and situations.
- Multiracial (ethnic, cultural) individuals have the right to claim membership in multiple identity groups.
- Multiracial (ethnic, cultural) individuals have the right to prioritize membership with one group over another.

Second, MRPs involved with student identity groups should work to avoid the trap of letting their groups be too internally focused. Although working outside of one's group to work with other groups takes additional time, resources, and planning, working with other identity groups not only promotes a larger understanding of identity among everyone in the group, but it also deals with the problems of either excluding or minimizing group members with multiple identities. One easy and efficient way for identity groups to cooperate with one another is through co-sponsorship. In co-sponsoring events, identity groups need to be clear about the responsibilities of each organization, such as advertising and food preparation. In this way, the groups encourage an infusion of new ideas and increase communication between the groups. The co-sponsoring groups also need to carefully balance the goals of their own group with those of the other group so that both groups benefit from the co-sponsoring experience.

An example of a co-sponsorship event might be the Black Sororities Union, the Women's Coalition, and the LGBT Alliance getting together to plan a panel of speakers during Women's History Month. Another co-sponsorship event might be one group inviting another group to attend one of their functions, such as the Islamic Student Group inviting Hillel (the Jewish student group) to the ending of Ramadan, the festival of Eid al-Fitr, and discussing the similarities and differences between the two religions' key festivals. Such a co-sponsorship event would not only increase understanding and appreciation between these two religions, but also benefit those multiple identity students who come from religiously mixed families.

Exercise for Improving Diversity Within Identity Groups

Identity groups, being naturally sensitive to issues of multiculturalism, might seem like odd places to promote even more diversity, but as we've seen in our discussion, there is room for improvement in making all students feel welcome within identity groups, in particular students with multiple identities. On the following list, put a check mark next to each item that you feel identity groups could do to facilitate increased diversity within identity groups, and put an "x" next to each item that is misguided in terms of increasing diversity within identity groups.

_____ **1.** Let students with multiple identities know that there is another group on campus that can help them explore that part of their identity.

_____ **2.** Organize regular get-togethers with a variety of other student identity organizations so that there is a consistent sense of interaction between groups.

_____ **3.** Make it clear in the organization's mission statements that many members of the group are in fact of multiple identities, and let all new members know that the organization is committed to talking about issues related to multiple identities.

_____ **4.** Refer students with multiple identities to the library, where they will find plentiful resources on multiple identity issues.

_____ **5.** Introduce students with similar multiple identities to each other and let them know that the college's administration probably won't fund such a specific organization so they should talk amongst themselves.

_____ **6.** Help to organize and/or support other campus organizations that already encompass students of multiple identities such as the Black and Latin LGBT Alliance.

_____ **7.** Suggest to students with multiple identities that they try entering counseling so that a trained professional can help them integrate their identities.

_____ **8.** Spend one meeting a year talking about multiple-identity issues.

_____ **9.** Provide multiple-identities books, DVDs, and pamphlets within the organization's meeting space, so that students from multiple identities feel supported in a variety of ways.

_____ **10.** Organize a multiple-identities awareness day, in which events and speakers focus on this specific topic.

As in previous exercises, sometimes the answers are less obvious than others, but in our estimation, the items that best demonstrate an identity group's commitment to recognizing the diversity of its own members are items 2, 3, 6, 9, and 10. The remaining items are less helpful because they treat multiple-identity issues as something to be discussed elsewhere (items 1 and 4), treat multiple-identity issues as if they are problematic and should be discussed privately or with a counselor (items 5 and 7), or pay only momentary lip service to the topic (item 8).

Finally, MRPs (again, whether or not they have multiple identities themselves), can follow action plans similar to the ones discussed in Chapter 2 to respond to the needs of students with multiple identities. Following are three sample action plans.

ACTION PLAN ONE: OBSERVATION (LEARNING FROM A SAFE DISTANCE)

Check each item you believe will help you reach your goals and in which you feel comfortable participating.

1. Watch films or television shows that deal with multiple identities such as *Secrets and Lies* and *A Family Thing* (both of which deal with biracial children and their families), *Brother to Brother* (about gay Black men), *Priest* (about a conflicted gay Catholic priest), and *Catfish in Black Bean Sauce* (about the Vietnamese adopted children of an African-American couple).

2. Do an Internet search on the words *multiracial* and *biracial* and explore some of the sites that come up.

3. Read one of the following books:
- *Stopping for Green Lights* by Alyce Miller
- *Color of our Future* by Farai Chideya
- *Twice Blessed: On Being Lesbian or Gay and Jewish* by Christie Balka
- *Caucasia* by Danzy Senna
- *Giovanni's Room* by James Baldwin

4. Keep a personal journal of your reactions and feelings to each one of the experiences.

ACTION PLAN TWO: INVESTIGATION (LEARNING FROM A CLOSER DISTANCE)

Select each of the items in which you would feel comfortable participating in and that you believe would assist you in achieving your personal growth goals:

1. Interview students with multiple identities.

2. Attend a variety of student identity group meetings (ask permission of those groups first), whether or not you identify with these groups. The variety should include a racial or ethnic identity group, a women's group, a religious group, and an LGBT group.

3. Join an online listserv dedicated to multiple-identity college students.

4. Continue to keep a journal of reactions and feelings generated from the experiences above.

ACTION PLAN THREE: DIRECT PARTICIPATION
(LEARNING FROM THE CLOSEST DISTANCE)

Select items from the following list that are comfortable for you and offer the greatest opportunity for growth and change.

1. Build on the friendships you initiated in the investigation phase by arranging to have dinner with a multiple-identity individual.

2. Arrange a co-sponsoring event. Talk with the president of each identity organization you attended and see if they would be interested in co-sponsoring with another identity organization.

3. Continue to keep a journal of reactions and feelings generated from the experiences above to be used as discussion topics for peers or significant others.

AWARENESS INTO ACTION: SURPASSING
OUT-OF-CLASSROOM VARIABLES

In this chapter, we attempt to demonstrate clearly the many ways in which students experience college and university life outside of the classroom in very different ways. Students may enter college with certain naive assumptions that all students will have the same experiences related to residence hall and Greek life, sports, extracurricular activities, and student identity groups, but the reality is that there are many variables to these aspects of college and university life, depending on who you are. As is the case with academic life on campus, awareness of the out-of-the-classroom variables students experience is the only way to respond to them positively. To become an MRP, become aware of the variables different people experience: different expectations about living with roommates and different experiences negotiating the Greek system; different and frequently biased experiences based on race, gender, and sexual orientation regarding college sports; different experiences involving privilege in relation to extracurricular activities; and different experiences with student identity groups, particularly for students who are LGBT, Arab or Muslim, or of multiple identities.

Despite roadblocks, however, students can learn a great deal from their out-of-class experiences in college. Becoming an MRP will be greatly facilitated by having a rich life outside of the classroom, not just by living and interacting within the residence halls, special-interest house, or fraternity/sorority, but also by becoming involved with campus organizations. Involvement in organizations has a long history of fostering multiculturally responsible action in people. Consider, for example, the story of Rosa Parks, who is often described as the "Mother of the Civil Rights Movement." Parks's refusal to move to the back of the bus on December 1, 1955 (which, if you are not familiar with the story, was the rule in segregated Montgomery, Alabama at the time), resulting first in the Montgomery Bus Boycott and eventually desegregation, was not simply a snap decision. Rather, Parks had spent 12 years helping lead the local NAACP chapter and had spent the previous summer attending a 10-day training session at a labor and civil rights organizing school, where she had met with members of an older generation of civil rights activists. In other words, Rosa Parks did not just come out of nowhere or single-handedly give birth to the civil rights movement. She was, in fact, part of an existing effort for change, which involved people striving to improve the world for all people.

CHAPTER AND PERSONAL REVIEW QUESTIONS

1. What are the four out-of-classroom variables that students of different races, ethnicities, cultures, and genders may experience?

2. What are some of the variables that students of different races, ethnicities, cultures, and genders may experience regarding housing (including fraternities and sororities)?

3. What are some of the variables that students of different races, ethnicities, cultures, and genders may experience regarding sports?

4. What are some of the variables that students of different races, ethnicities, cultures, and genders may experience regarding extracurricular activities?

5. What are some of the variables that students of different races, ethnicities, cultures, and genders may experience regarding identity groups?

6. What is the difference between Arabs and Muslims? Have you ever confused the terms? Explain.

7. What is the definition of *multiple identities*?

8. What are the five stages of Poston's Bicultural Development Model and what are the characteristics of each stage?

9. What are the six points of Root's Multiracial Bill of Rights? How do these six points apply to people who are not multiracial but do have other multiple identities?

10. Now that you have learned about the ways racially, ethnically, and culturally diverse students, as well as women, experience housing and extracurricular life differently from men and/or those in the majority groups, are you motivated to help make changes in these areas? Why or why not? If yes, what steps do you plan to take?

REFERENCES

Kivel, P. (2002). *Uprooting racism: How white people can work for racial justice* (Rev. ed.). British Columbia: Canada: New Society Publishers.

Poston, W. S. C. (1990). The Biracial identity development model. *Journal of Counseling and Development, 69,* 152–155.

Root, M. P. (1992). *Racially mixed people in America.* Newbury Park: Sage Publications.

CHAPTER 6

▲▲▲
▼▼▼

Understanding and Establishing Multicultural Relationships

BEFORE YOU READ

1. In your college experience, have you considered the potential benefits of not just attending class and completing assignments, but also developing mentoring relationships with professors and other college staff? Why or why not?

2. How important are friendships to you in your college experience? Do you focus mainly on your studies and consider friendships to be secondary to your studies, or do you consider friendships to be intrinsic to the college experience? If the former, please explain why you feel that way? If the latter, how important is it to you to foster friendships with individuals from different racial, ethnic, and cultural groups, as well as members of different genders? Please explain why you feel that way?

3. How receptive are you to developing relationships with people from races and/or ethnicities other than your own? Please explain why you feel that way?

4. Whether or not you are yourself lesbian, gay, or bisexual, how comfortable are you with lesbian, gay, and bisexual intimate relationships? Please explain why you feel that way?

5. How aware are you of the various power imbalances that can occur in all types of relationships? Are you aware of abuses of power, such as emotional and psychological abuse, physical abuse, sexual assault, acquaintance rape, and date rape? How would you define and differentiate these terms?

INTRODUCTION

B eyond academics (discussed in Chapter 4) and housing/extracurricular activities (discussed in Chapter 5), what would the college experience be if there were no mentoring relationships between faculty, staff, and students; friendships among peers; and intimate relationships? Interactions among faculty, peers, and intimate partners are a large part of the college experience. Many students will have lived relatively homogeneous existences prior to entering college, unless they have lived in diverse neighborhoods and/or gone to diverse high schools. Students who have had enriching experiences with diversity prior to entering college may have a head start becoming multiculturally responsible persons (MRPs). Students who have not had diverse pre-college experiences should consider the college experience an opportunity to meet individuals different from themselves. Among the myriad of relationships that exist on college campuses, cross-racial, cross-ethnic, and cross-cultural relationships provide excellent opportunities for growth and practice in participating in a multicultural world beyond college.

A great deal can be learned from healthy multicultural relationships. The more attention students devote to positive multicultural relationships in college, the more likely they are to initiate multicultural contacts and build multicultural alliances essential for community growth and development in the post-college world. In this chapter we will explore various types of relationships students may develop in college and examine some of the pitfalls of these relationships in an effort to help MRPs better understand the problems and move beyond them. Each of the primary types of college relationships—mentoring relationships with professors and other college staff, friendships, and intimate relationships—will be examined.

BUILDING MENTORING RELATIONSHIPS WITH PROFESSORS AND OTHER COLLEGE STAFF

There is general agreement that relationships between students and college personnel are valuable. As a mentor, the faculty member, graduate teaching assistant, coach, librarian, academic advisor, administrator, or departmental staff member can provide individualized support and care, and facilitate the development of a young person's dreams. Such mentors serve as role models who guide, tutor, and perform the role of confidant. In addition, mentors can share valued skills, broaden students' perspectives, support students' academic pursuits, promote student involvement in campus life, encourage personal growth, and multicultural awareness.

Unfortunately, a large number of college students go through their entire college experience without forming a significant mentor/mentee relationship with anyone. Several of the reasons for this will be discussed briefly: First, many classes are so large and/or departments so busy that it is not practical for professors or other staff members to establish mentoring relationships with students. Second, many professors focus more on didactic content in their teaching than on the interpersonal dynamics between themselves and students. In addition, other staff members such as teaching assistants and departmental staff may not see mentoring individual students as part of their jobs. Third, students who are less assertive than others do not believe that they have the right to infringe on or impose their need for mentoring upon their professors or other staff. Fourth, many students are not aware of the fact that relationships between themselves and their professors/staff are possible. Fifth—and here is where a multicultural-oriented roadblock presents itself—sometimes racial/ethnic/cultural identity statuses (discussed in Chapter 2) between professors/staff members and students do not match. For example, at one college, a major conflict erupted when a White advisor of an African-American student said, "If I had anything to do with it, Blacks would no do research on Blacks and females would no do research on females." Clearly, the relationship between this student and academic advisor was debilitative and was unlikely to promote personal growth. Another debilitative relationship would probably occur when the professor or staff member and the student have

---

REFLECTION

Do you have mentor/mentee relationships with any of your instructors? How about other staff members on campus such as advisors, coaches, departmental staff members, and members of the library staff? If you do not, why not? If you do, what actions did you and/or your mentors take to develop those relationships?

DEFINITION

Dyads. As described by Helms (1984), *dyads* are the relationships that occur in a counseling situation—and by extension in a mentor/mentee situation—that are based on the racial/ethnic identity development statuses. There are four types of dyads: In a **progressive** dyad, the mentor's identity status is at least one level higher than that of the mentee (e.g., the mentor is at the integrative awareness stage and the mentee is at the internalization stage), and the mentor is therefore able to facilitate growth in the mentee. In a **parallel** dyad, the mentor and mentee see the world in the same way and so the mentor will be unlikely to help facilitate growth in the mentee. In a **regressive** dyad, the mentee's racial/cultural identity development is at a higher stage than that of the mentor, which results in an unproductive relationship between mentor and mentee. Finally, in a **crossed** dyad, the mentor and mentee are diametrically opposed in their views regarding race/ethnicity/culture, resulting in an emotionally charged and unproductive relationship.

directly opposite racial/ethnic/cultural identity attitudes, otherwise known as crossed dyads.

There are several things students can do to facilitate relationships with professors and other potentially mentoring staff members, such as introducing themselves, showing respect to potential mentors in terms of their positions and workload, and asking questions.

ESTABLISHING AND MAINTAINING HEALTHY FRIENDSHIPS

Among the wide variety of activities in which college students become engaged upon arrival at college, establishing and maintaining friendships is one of the most important. Students tend to select friends who are similar to themselves in terms of their racial/ethnic/cultural identities, values, perspectives, political affiliations, religious orientation, and special interests. Although establishing friendships based on similarities is often the most comfortable way to initiate friendly relationships, it is not necessarily the most growth enhancing. Students are encouraged to take advantage of a time in their lives when they are in the position of being around a wide array of diverse people. After college, unless individuals live and work in diverse communities or choose professions that attract diverse employees, people tend to gravitate back to the environments from which they came, and so the cycle of little interaction with people from groups other than their own may continue throughout life. The opportunity to break that cycle exists on the college campus. Most colleges attract students from a wide array of racial, ethnic, and cultural backgrounds and from nations all around the world. The environment provides an oasis for potential cross-cultural friendships, because not only do students of many different identities coexist on college campuses, but they also are placed in a position where they are much more likely to interact in the classroom, in residence halls, at social events, in sports, and in extracurricular activities than they might be after college. Colleges and universities can become an educational launching pad, preparing students to live and thrive in an increasingly multicultural and globally focused world. Choosing to be a part of that multicultural, global world when the opportunity is there, can be an advantage to one's life and career.

The first step in diversifying your friendships is to assess the level of diversity among the friends you already have. After that, developing inter-racial/ethnic/cultural friendships will involve a high level of awareness, respect, and the ability to have difficult conversations. However, it is worth the effort because it is through multicultural friendships that individuals can gain an internalized understanding of cultural diversity that reading books and magazines and watching films can only partly provide.

Exercise for Assessing the Diversity of Your Friendships

DIRECTIONS: Please answer the following questions and discuss your responses to these questions with a classmate or friend.

1. How similar or different are the socioeconomic statuses of your friends in comparison to your socioeconomic status?

2. How similar to or different from your sexual orientation are their sexual orientations?

3. How similar to or different from your racial/ethnic identity are their racial/ethnic identities?

4. Are the religious backgrounds of any of your friends different from your own?

5. Are any of your friends living with a disability?

6. Do you maintain friendships with members of both sexes or primarily with members of your own sex?

7. Do any of your friends identify as transgender or genderqueer?

8. On a scale of 1 to 10 (1 = low and 10 = high), how much diversity exists among your closest friends?

9. Do your friends challenge your perspectives regarding diversity?

10. To what extent are you satisfied and comfortable with the level of diversity among your friends?

Initiating communication with strangers can be challenging and scary, especially when the strangers are from groups different from your own—groups with which you have had little or no prior interaction. There are many hindering forces to multicultural communication. One such hindering force is stereotyping. Stereotyping is a process through which individual qualities are ignored and are not respected. When internalized, stereotyping can be a major threat to personal growth and to multicultural communication and interaction. A second hindering force can be different racial, ethnic, and cultural identity statuses. We suggest that multicultural connections can be made between students by adapting Helms's model of social dyads. As discussed earlier in this chapter, Helms's dyad model suggests that certain dyad types promote harmony between individuals (parallel or progressive), while other dyad types promote discord (regressive or crossed). Those in parallel dyads will have similar worldviews and will place about the same emphasis on race, ethnicity, and/or culture. Therefore, the individuals may not only be comfortable initiating a conversation, but may progress toward building an ongoing, harmonious relationship. For those in progressive dyads, one of the individuals would be slightly more advanced regarding racial, ethnic, and/or cultural identity status than the other, but the relationship can still work, because the individual at the less progressive identity status can learn from the individual who is at the more progressive identity status without being too far behind. For those in a regressive dyad, one individual will be significantly more advanced in racial, ethnic, and/or cultural identity status, resulting in a conflicted relationship that may not work. Likewise, those in crossed dyads would be conflicted and probably will not develop a friendship, because their identity statuses are diametrically opposed (e.g., one individual is in the conflict stage and feels that race is unimportant while the other individual is in the autonomy stage and believes not only that race is essential but also that actively working to relinquish racism is a priority). In short, in order for communication to occur and for friendships to develop out of communication, both individuals must share a common worldview and a common goal. In the crossed dyad, for instance, alliances are difficult, if not impossible, to reach because each member of the dyad believes that the other is essentially wrong in his or her worldview or perspective.

Exercise for Putting the Dyad Model Into Practice

Let's imagine four women who meet in their college orientation class for the first time: Amy is a young woman who has had major conflicts with her sisters and with other females in high school. She tends to distrust other women, would not refer to herself as a feminist, and chooses to be closer to males. Barbara has a close relationship with her male fraternal twin. She tends to have more male friends than female friends. Cindy is an only child and has a large group of male and female friends. She is outgoing and enjoys interacting with a wide range of individuals. Debra tends to be introverted and likes to maintain a small group of friends. She has recently become involved in a women's political organization, and during high school she helped organize events for Women's History Month.

Amy and Barbara are a parallel dyad, as are Cindy and Debra. The individuals in these two dyads will possess similar worldviews and may build harmonious relationships. However, it is unlikely that Amy and Barbara will challenge one another to become more multiculturally responsible, because they are both similar. Now that you have an idea of how gender can be applied to the dyad model, please answer the following questions:

1. Which dyads reflect a progressive relationship? What could the woman who is more advanced in her identity status do to help the other person become more multiculturally responsible?

2. Which dyads reflect a regressive relationship? What could the more multiculturally advanced individual do to help the other person become more aware? How could power limit growth?

3. Which dyads reflect a crossed relationship? How might each individual feel minimized or judged? What could each individual do to assist the other in growth?

We suggest that you begin to explore development of culturally diverse friendships with individuals who you believe are more advanced in their racial/ethnic/cultural identity status than yourself, or who are parallel with you—and then work from there. Because all people share something in common, we encourage you to use common experiences and interests (e.g., similar interests in films, common places traveled to, shared hobbies) as starting points for communication and interaction. Progressing to talking to friends about diversity issues can be challenging. However, regardless of your racial/ethnic/cultural identity or that of potential friends, it is a challenge worth taking on as an MRP.

UNDERSTANDING INTIMATE RELATIONSHIPS

Interracial and Interethnic Dating

If creating diverse friendships can feel like hiking up a mountain, interracial and interethnic dating can feel like climbing Mount Everest. Challenges to inter-cultural dating come from family and from the racial or ethnic groups of both individuals in the relationship.

The issues of interracial and interethnic dating are not new. In terms of popular culture, as far back as 1915 the controversial D.W. Griffith film *Birth of a Nation* depicted in racist terms the supposed dangers of miscegenation (the mixing of races) in a female character who leaps to her death rather than surrender to the advances of an escaped Negro slave. In 1927, the Broadway production of *Showboat* depicted in now-dated terms issues related to interracial couples. In the musical, a performer on the *Cotton Blossom* showboat, Julie LaVerne, is a successful lead singer. However, Julie and her husband Steve are forced to leave the showboat when it is revealed that Julie has "Negro" blood in her, breaking then-existing laws about interracial marriage. The issue of interracial dating between White men and Asian women was the topic of the 1957 film *Sayonara*. The film tells the story of American servicemen in Japan during the Korean War, several of whom fall in love with Japanese women. In the film, one interracial couple commits double suicide rather than face censure from both Japanese society and the U.S. Army.

These examples from older films may seem melodramatic and even silly to us today, but for many people the issue of interracial and interethnic dating and marriage is still controversial. Consider, for example, some films that explore interracial and interethnic relationships in a more contemporary way. These films do not go so far as to have the characters involved in "mixed" relationships melodramatically commit suicide as a result of societal pressures, but the films do still have "controversial" written all over them. As long ago as 1967, the film *Guess Who's Coming to Dinner* was the film that broke the mold by dealing with interracial relationships in a more adult manner than had been attempted before in films. The movie depicts the reaction of both sets of parents of a young interracial couple, who spend a long, difficult evening working through their reactions to the announcement that their children want to get married. While still very relevant in some ways, the film is also dated in the overly delicate, class-conscious way it approaches the subject of a Black man and a White woman announcing their engagement. In the film the rosiest picture imaginable is painted of the couple, with the White woman as the eternal "colorblind" optimist and the Black man as a doctor who lives in Switzerland (as if to suggest that an average Black man might not be an acceptable mate for a White woman, but an upper-class Black man would be). Still, the film broke new ground and coincided with the Supreme Court's declaration that laws prohibiting interracial marriage were unconstitutional. At that time, 16 states still had laws prohibiting interracial marriage. It was not until 2000 that the last state to overturn the law, Alabama, finally did so.

Since the 1990s, such films as *Mississippi Masala*, *Save the Last Dance*, and *My Big Fat Greek Wedding* have reflected the times in which they were made by showing that, while American society is now more accepting of interracial and interethnic relationships (which was not the case at the time of *Guess Who's Coming to Dinner*), such relationships are still controversial within communities and families. For instance, *Mississippi Masala* depicts the relationship between a Black man and an Indian-American woman, which causes intense friction between the man's and the woman's families. Although played for laughs, one of the key themes in *My Big Fat Greek Wedding* is the controversy in the family of the main character, Toula, over her dating and potentially marrying a man who is not Greek like them.

> **REFLECTION**
>
> Are you involved in an interracial or interethnic relationship? Or do you know anyone who is involved in such a relationship? Even if you are not or do not know anyone personally who is involved in such a relationship, how difficult do you think it is for both parties in such relationships? Why do you think that is the case?

Perhaps the most discussed form of mixed relationship that still generates the most friction is the interracial relationship between a Black man and a White woman or between a Black woman and a White man. From the early development of the United States to the present, the overall attitude toward Black and White interracial dating has been overwhelmingly negative. The perception is that when a White woman dates a Black male, she gives up her "whiteness," and he, in turn rejects his "blackness." The end result is that the couple ends up breaking taboos emanating from both White society and Black society (she is rejecting her White privilege and he is reaching toward White privilege at the expense of the Black women he could be dating). The same could be said of Black women who date White men.

In 1991, Spike Lee commented on Black/White relationships in his movie *Jungle Fever,* in which a successful Black architect and an Italian-American temp worker get together, resulting in much animosity from both families. Interestingly, in this film, Spike Lee chooses to make the Black character successful and the White Italian-American character not so successful (and, it should be noted that the situation is complicated by the fact that the interracial affair is extramarital and her Italian-American ethnicity removes her somewhat from White privilege, which is largely held by those from Anglo backgrounds). Nonetheless, the same perceptions about White privilege versus Black rejection of race present themselves. He is seen as rejecting his African-American culture and she is seen as rejecting both her White privilege and her Italian-American ethnicity.

Ten years later, in the film *Save the Last Dance*, a White girl is transferred to a Chicago school that is comprised mostly of Black students. The White girl, Sara, begins dating a Black male, Derek. Although most members of both families seem to be supportive of this arrangement, there is one critical incident in the movie in which Derek's sister, Chenille, challenges Sara, saying that Sara is stealing one of the few Black men in their school who is likely to be very successful, thereby taking away a Black man from the Black women at the school. So, even in a film in which a Black and White interracial relationship is accepted by most of the characters, controversy is still not completely out of the picture.

What does all this film history have to do with interracial and interethnic dating on college campuses? The connection is simply that interracial and interethnic dating is still likely to raise some eyebrows, and students involved in interracial and interethnic relationships should be prepared for an uphill battle. Perceptions that White people only date Black people because Black people are viewed as more sexually adventurous, or that Black people date White people to "lighten" their social standing (e.g., make themselves more "White" somehow), or that non-Jews date Jews to potentially earn positions of financial comfort, or that Asian people date outside of their race to avoid the perspective that Asians are overly academic and "uncool," or that Hispanic people date Black people because they are both from rough, urban backgrounds are all based on racial and ethnic stereotypes. But these stereotypes persist nonetheless and may lead to misunderstanding, confrontation, harassment, or even violence. Consider, for example, the following incidents that have occurred on campuses in recent years:

- In 1997, three people wearing ski masks threatened a student at a large university in the Midwest because he was a White male walking a Black woman to her dorm room.

- Bob Jones University in South Carolina rescinded its ban on interracial relationships only after a highly publicized visit to the campus from George W. Bush in 2000, which resulted in a public outcry when President Bush failed to comment on the ban.

- In 2001, at the University of Mississippi, a White male had two pieces of asphalt hurled through his residence hall window. Attached was a note saying, "You're going to get it, you Godforsaken nigger-lover." The next night, someone tried to set his door on fire.

The incidents in the preceding list are extreme examples of nonacceptance of interracial and interethnic relationships. On a more personal and typical scale, consider the following experience of Renee, an African-American woman who has dated two White men: Brian (for a brief period of time) and then Ian (for several years).

When I started writing this I thought I was going to completely focus on my relationship with Ian. But then I realized that I had to discuss a bit of my relationship with Brian if only for the reason that, brief as it was, I also learned some things from that time with Brian. I applied those lessons with Brian to my relationship with Ian; some things worked and some did not.

I was not the most confident person when I was dating Brian, which I think led to our breaking up. That's neither here nor there, but the important thing was that by the time I dated Ian, there were things that I would not put up with because I had learned my lesson with Brian. Eventually with Ian I became more vocal, more demanding, and I spent more time thinking about my issues with race.

I would suggest you discuss your issues/baggage/whatever about race up front. Because the issues exist, and ignoring them will not make them go away. And you might as well take this time to figure out what personal "demons" you have about race while you're having that discussion with your partner. Preferably before.

When dating Brian, I was perfectly aware that I was breaking some "taboos" there but I really did not discuss them with Brian because I thought I was above it, and he was above it, and anyone who had a problem with seeing a White man dating a Black woman was just a racist pig. Wrong. Pretending that issues of race are not there is stupid. Denying your race is stupid. Not discussing that your dating is going to make people you do not even know uncomfortable, possibly opening you up to ridicule and scorn, is stupid. Get the picture? If two people of different races even think that their dating, relationship, or whatever is going to become serious, they need to talk about what they're going to face out in the real world. Because even in our enlightened twenty-first-century age, you are going to face some nasty stuff if you date outside your race. Better to face it up front than to have it bite you in the behind.

Brian and I never really had fights or disagreements about race; but we did not have discussions about it either. I remember distinctly during that time feeling like I was "getting away with something" by dating Brian. It goes back to breaking those taboos and feeling like you're doing something rebellious or scandalous because you can. Now that sounds infantile, but at the time I was young and inexperienced. My point here is that folks should not get involved in an interracial relationship because it's "taboo," "exotic," or "on the edge." When I think about the many people in the past who were beaten or harassed or terrorized because of an interracial relationship, it makes me wonder what people who do this sort of thing "casually" are thinking.

Anyway, I did not discuss any of my feelings or thoughts with Brian (and he did not discuss his with me), so whatever uncomfortable feelings we had about our race (and our religion) did not get out in the open. And I felt tension because of that. By the time I met Ian, not only did I want to discuss it all the time, I probably beat it into the ground. But that's another discussion.

I remember distinctly that when Ian and I were out in public (eating, shopping, whatever) we got stares from people who saw us. And trust me, they were not all gaga because we were so in love with each other. You know that living in Florida is sometimes like living in the Deep South of the 1950s and 1960s. There were older Whites and Blacks who were uncomfortable seeing an interracial couple in public. I remember getting dirty looks. I remember being ignored by waiters and waitresses. I remember being treated like a non-person simply because I chose to date a White man (and he chose to date a Black woman). He and I used to discuss this all the time. We could not simply go out to breakfast on a Sunday morning and read the paper and drink coffee like everybody else. Because of other people's attitudes and biases, it became a political statement, and it affected what we did and sometimes where we went. And we talked about that. I cannot stress how much of a good thing this was. It led us to not only discover the nature of our relationship, but also to figure out our own personal beliefs and biases, and what was true and was not. Sometimes we became closer from it; sometimes there were shouting matches.

One of the worst fights was when I accused him of being a racist (over what issue I have no idea . . . probably because of one of the many silly disagreements we had about politics). He was livid. He literally punched a wall and stormed out of our apartment in the middle of the night. I did not hear from him for hours and I called a friend in a panic because I did not know where the man was. That separation gave me a lot of time to think, and by the time Ian returned I realized that it was me who was projecting my racist issues about Whites on him. I apologized and he apologized and we worked on rebuilding trust. But it was important that we had that fight, to get whatever issue we had out in the open. Communication is the key in any relationship, but especially in interracial relationships.

So I meet Ian, we start digging each other, and things start getting serious. We moved in with each other and we started talking marriage. Marriage means family. And that's where a lot of our problems began. A lot of times interracial relationships fail not because of the two people involved, but because of their respective families. If you're dating someone of a different race, tell your family up front, whether you think they're going to be upset or not.

I knew early on when I met Ian that I wanted our relationship to be a serious, lasting one. I think early on I knew that I wanted to marry him. When we reached that point in our relationship where we were talking about moving in with each other and using the future tense in all of our sentences, I told my mother about Ian. And I told her that he was White.

I did not expect her to accept him, and she did not. As a matter of fact, for the longest time she did not acknowledge his existence. She forbade me to move in with him, and when I did, she did not ask about him and did not speak to him. For a long time, she did not even refer to him to by name. It was a long hard road getting her to accept him. She made it clear to me that I was choosing a difficult path by choosing to date someone of another race, especially a White man. Even though she did not say it, I felt she was disappointed in me for not choosing a Black man because she felt that I did not think they were good enough. Maybe she had her own issues for helping to foster that belief in me. In any event, she reminded me often of how difficult it was going to be to be in an interracial relationship. And although it took her a long time to come around, I think what facilitated that was the fact that I was honest with her and let her know what was happening from the "get-go," so to speak.

One of the biggest setbacks Ian and I had was two weeks before I was to meet his mother and sisters for the first time, which was when he told me that he had not told his mom that I was Black. All this time he had been calling his mother weekly (as was his habit) and writing his father in Chicago (as was his habit) and he had not told them that I was Black. I think he was going to spring this on his mom when I met her; who knows when he intended to tell his father. As you can imagine, I hit the roof.

There is nothing more disheartening to find out than that your partner has hidden something from you or lied to you . . . but it's even worse when it involves race. What that action told me was that Ian was ashamed of me and ashamed of my race. Ian not discussing my race with his family made me feel inferior and put me in a position where it was going to be even harder to win their trust and respect. During our entire relationship I bent over backwards to make inroads with his mother, at one time believing that his family accepted me.

If someone of your family has a problem with your partner's race, it's better to let them know. Be ready to engage. And more important, be prepared to disagree with your family if your relationship is that important to you.

Like I said before, my mother did not accept Ian at first. I let him know that. I also let him know that our relationship was important enough to me to endure my mother's criticism and her ostracism. But I also made it clear that I was attempting to change her mind about him. I tried to never let him think that it was okay with me that my mother did not accept him. It was okay for her to disagree with me about Ian, but it was not okay for her to be disagreeable and disrespectful toward him. Again, it comes back to respect. I'm not saying that people need to come to blows with their loved ones over their relationship, but you better be sure that they know that you will not accept anything but respectful behavior toward your partner. Your family does not get to treat your partner like a second-class citizen because of his or her race.

I found very late into the game that Ian's mother did not accept our relationship, although she had said she did (something like two or three years after we first started seeing each other and after we were engaged). As a matter of fact, she told Ian that she was simply waiting for us to break up before she mentioned how she had never liked me and thought our interracial relationship was "not natural" (her words). Ian did not know any of this; like me he had taken his mother's word that I was accepted as his girlfriend, and eventually, fiancée. When he found out that she had lied to him, he really did not know how to take it. What he never did, which I pushed him to do often, was to defend me and defend our relationship. I think I forgave him for that, but I'm still not sure after all this time if I ever trusted him after that.

It is extremely important to have "allies" within your family and friends. It will make your life much easier. Both Ian and I found our allies in the most unlikely of places. Ian's ally became his father. Initially, his father did not approve of our relationship (even urging Ian in a letter to "satisfy his curiosity" about me and move on), but once he met me he changed his mind. We were even a bit friendly after Ian and I broke up. But because Ian had someone in his family who supported our relationship and made efforts to discuss race, it made it easier for him to, in the short run, discuss these contentious issues with his mother.

My allies came in the form of my father and maternal grandmother. I was surprised that when she met Ian she took to him rather quickly and endorsed our relationship. She urged me to stay with Ian if it made me happy, despite the objections from my mother and other members of my family. She reminded me that it was my life to live, and that no one was in any position to judge another's actions or decisions. I took that advice to heart every time I discussed my relationship with Ian with my mother. Because I did not back down I think my mother realized I really cared for him, and eventually she chose to accept him.

I have to say that my personal friends (and to my knowledge his friends) were wholly supportive of our relationship. I certainly did not witness or notice any animosity or racist attitudes from any of our immediate friends. I did not witness a lot of animosity coming from other students, or maybe more accurately said, I did not notice it. But admittedly, I did not have a lot of Black friends when I was in college. I was not involved in African-American culture during college. I am sure things would have been a lot different if I were, and perhaps I would never have gotten involved with Brian or Ian. Either way, I think my fellow students and friends were more amazed that Ian and I got engaged at 20 than that we were of different races.

I cannot say that I regret what came out of those relationships, even though I'm not with either Brian or Ian now. Both relationships have contributed to making me the person I am, as with all life experiences. Things ended with Ian so badly that we have not seen or spoken with each other in over 10 years. There are times when I wonder what's happened to Ian, but not enough to track him down and certainly not enough to ever let him back into my life again. Because issues with his family were so poorly handled (and because of his own personal issues) I do not think I could ever be friends with him again. I simply could not trust him again.

Ironically, Brian and I still talk to each other. After not seeing each other for 10 years, we've managed to track each other down, and for two people living on opposite coasts, we've kept in decent contact with each other. I wonder what would have happened if I had met Brian after Ian or if I had met him at another phase in my life. I often refer to Brian as "the one who got away," never really wanting to deeply explore why he got away. I do not think I'll ever be happy with my level of naiveté at that time in my life.

As Renee has stated, she is no longer in contact with Ian because the relationship ended poorly. However, she is still in touch with Brian. By way of comparison, consider Brian's account of his relationship with Renee:

To be honest, interracial dating has never been that big an issue for me. Physical appearance as a whole doesn't matter to me. I tend to go for gleams in the eye, intelligence, how a woman carries herself, that sort of thing. However, during my one interracial dating experience, I do have to confess that there was a slight concern on my part. Not anything intrinsic, but more a concern of how it might "appear."

By way of background: Renee was the second girl I had ever dated, ever. I was a late bloomer of sorts and had only dated one girl in high school. Once I got to college, I was still emotionally involved with said high school sweetheart, so I did not exactly start with the ladies right away. Renee and I met at a college function organized by the residence halls and hit it off. We started doing "freshman dating," which is that peculiar sort of dating where you do not actually go out anywhere but hang out in dorm rooms with friends and sometimes "mess around."

Interracial dating is going to challenge your stereotypes about different races and cultures. It is important to be open to these lessons so the relationship can progress. Her race never really stopped me from being with her. I mean, when you get down to it, "black skin" is more a signifier than anything else, some sort of icon detached from reality. If a person is Black, that person is supposed to be certain things, and Renee was a lesson that, er, no, that's not quite the case. For example, she's a Sting fan—a huuuuuuge, drooly Sting fan. When you think of a "Black female" I would guess that

"Sting fan" is not one of the stereotypical attributes you would think of. So there was that little lesson for me.

Everything about you will determine how a relationship progresses: your interests, your culture, your family, and your dating experience and maturity level—especially the maturity level. This, of course, is in addition to your comfort with race and the racial/cultural identity of both people.

On the other hand, I do have to confess that as a horribly insecure 18-year-old with extremely limited experience. I was super-conscious about "what people might think" about Renee and me. This was not so much what you would expect; I was fantastically preoccupied with how people would judge me with any woman, especially friends. I am not sure if this is common among insecure young men—if it is, that's only comforting in that we are all inexperienced. So *every* potential girlfriend was held up to impossible scrutiny as I searched for reasons to be embarrassed by her. "Oh, my friends might think she's overweight." "Oh, my friends won't think she's funny." "Oh, she's not attractive enough for my group." So in my mind at the time, Renee's race became a reason to stay distant or not to get too attached. Insofar as race was a factor, that was the extent of it.

Except for those who are currently in an interracial relationship, the cultural issues are something to be dealt with "later." This means that people may sometimes be surprised or challenged when they enter into interracial or intercultural relationships.

REFLECTION

Discuss the differences between Renee's and Brian's stories. How are they similar? How do their racial identities affect their worldview? Although neither Renee nor Brian discusses religion at length, they do both mention it. To what extent might religious differences affect a relationship, interracial or not? How might the stories be different if Renee were Asian American and Brian were Native American? How might their stories be the same?

I can see race only being a factor in any future relationship insofar as it speaks to cultural differences: You come from this world, I come from mine, will the two intersect in a meaningful way? But that happens with any person. Now, if I were to bring a Black woman home to my parents, that might be a bit disconcerting for them at first, as I'm theoretically supposed to marry a nice Jewish girl. Also, my dad will make the occasional horribly inappropriate "joke" that makes me cringe in that full-body way.

But that would be a bridge to be crossed much farther down the road. And, frankly, who I date, sleep with, or marry is not their concern.

It is very clear that even in relationships, people will be in different places. Renee is aware of her race at every moment, while Brian focuses on his own personal growth and does not spend much time thinking about Renee's race. A review of the section on racial identity status will help you understand Renee's and Brian's positions regarding the importance of race. A review of the identity dyads discussed earlier in this chapter will give you an idea of whether their relationship was facilitative or debilitative.

Exercise for Determining Your Feelings About Interracial and Interethnic Dating

DIRECTIONS: Given that you have now been exposed to interracial dating through a discussion of popular culture (movies) and the personal dialogues of Renee and Brian, please respond to the following questions, paying attention to your immediate emotional reactions.

1. What racial make-up do you think of when you hear the phrase "interracial dating" (e.g., White/Black, Asian/Hispanic, etc.)? What ethnicities do you think of when you hear the phase "interethnic dating" (Italian American, Hispanic American, Jewish American, etc.)?

2. What is your reaction to a White male dating a Black female?

3. What is your reaction to a Black male dating a White female? How is this different from your reaction to question 2?

4. What is your reaction to Black people and Hispanic-American people dating each other? Is that reaction different than your reaction to Black and White people dating each other? Please explain.

5. Have any of your friends dated interracially and/or interethnically? What was your first reaction to those relationships? If you have had no such personal experience, what is your perception of how you would react to a friend dating interracially and/or interethnically?

6. Have you dated interracially or interethnically? What was that experience like? If you have not, what is your perception of how it would be?

7. Have you ever wanted to date interracially or interethnically but chose not to because of stigma or societal pressure?

8. Do you believe that interracial/interethnic dating is a good thing or not? Please explain.

Discuss your answers with people with whom you feel comfortable, and devise an action plan for you and your friends to deal with this potential issue.

As an MRP, it is important for you to examine your own thoughts and beliefs regarding interracial and interethnic dating and to increase your understanding of the challenges to interracial dating. Such an activity would assist you toward becoming a more multiculturally responsible individual.

Same-Sex and Bisexual Relationships

Interracial and intercultural relationships are not the only types of relationships that may feel like climbing Mount Everest. Whether or not you are yourself lesbian, gay, or bisexual, or know someone who is, imagine the difficulties such couples experience on campus. As the following account from Matthew—a gay student—shows, same-sex dating at college can be a complicated and sometimes frightening experience.

<table>
<tr><td>

REFLECTION

If you are a straight student who has been or is currently in a relationship, take a moment to consider some of the things you take for granted. Do you tell all of your friends that you are in a new relationship? Do you hold hands or kiss your partner in public? Now put that in perspective by comparing it with the experiences of lesbian, gay, and bisexual students. How do the experiences compare?

</td></tr>
</table>

I have dated in college, out in the real world, and now again in graduate school. My relationships have always been affected by my age as well as by the developmental stage of my partner. When I was a freshman in college I met and fell for a junior. We first got together during inebriated and unwise circumstances. Basically, we decided to have sex in my dorm shower and were caught and subsequently threatened by my dorm mates. It sure is not easy living in an apartment with five other guys who want you to leave, or perhaps even die. It was important to me in principle to stay in the dorm until the end of the semester to show them that they could not intimidate me.

My first boyfriend and I were openly gay pretty much everywhere we went. Back then we were practically a symbol of gay liberation personified. However, as open as we were all over town and campus, my boyfriend was not out to his parents, and I felt like I was his dirty little secret. My parents knew I was gay and met my boyfriend a few times. They were not especially happy about my being gay, but even then I think they knew that my policy was that I insisted on my relationships being treated as seriously as my sister's relationships. The double life has never suited me. Neither has kowtowing (submitting) to public opinion when I thought it was wrong.

I have been openly gay and openly affectionate with all of my partners since my first dating experience. I am very clear about my expectations of my partners—I ain't hiding for nobody! There are consequences for this attitude, though. I have been called names and accosted an uncountable number of times. I have been threatened with violence. In graduate school I had the door to my apartment vandalized with homophobic graffiti. I have had my life threatened verbally on more than one occasion. Every time I engage in public displays of affection with my partner I am aware of the risk of harassment and violence. Kisses and hugs are dangerous. It is mentally draining to have to do a risk assessment when I want to express spontaneous affection. Not only do I have to consider if it will be dangerous to my partner and me, but I also have to consider whether my affection is going to make my partner feel vulnerable. It makes me angry, if I let it, that I cannot engage in the same public behaviors as my classmates without fearing physical harm. When safety and principle are put in opposition to each other and partners come down on opposite sides of the struggle it can be a real challenge to the relationship. I am not sure if I have ever seen casual same-sex affection on campus outside of a specifically gay context.

Negotiating this with a potential boyfriend for the first time is really awkward. "I really like you, but are you willing to risk public harassment and possibly violence to be with me as openly as heterosexuals are with each other?" If the two of you are at different levels of comfort with your sexuality, it gets more difficult.

Family offers another challenge, as mentioned above. When one partner is out to his family and the other isn't, guess who is going to be feeling rejected during the holidays. If the family knows about the relationship and rejects it, that also puts a strain on the relationship. Defending your relationship to your family can be mentally and emotionally exhausting. Defending yourself to your partner for not defending your relationship to your family can be just as exhausting. Fortunately, some families really are accepting. My parents got there eventually, but it was not an easy road.

Heterosexual friends can usually only understand your challenges intellectually. They rarely can understand how it feels to always be under attack. You can hardly go a day without hearing an anti-gay comment somewhere— especially on college campuses. If you are open and confident in your sexuality, then your friends have even more difficulty understanding the frustration of constantly being invalidated both as a person and as a member of a relationship.

Finding a gay community to accept you is sometimes your best bet. At least there you do not have to explain or justify yourself all the time. Nor do you have to spend time educating your friends about why you are the way you are—and that goes far beyond simply why you are gay.

As Matthew's story indicates, students who are or want to be in lesbian, gay, or bisexual same-sex relationships have a lot of hurdles with which to deal. In Matthew's case, he has surmounted (perhaps to his danger) the two major obstacles, which are the choices as to whether or not to be open about your relationships and whether or not to display spontaneous affection publicly. Many students are not at Matthew's level of comfort or confidence when they enter college (or even when they leave college). Incidents of harassment and intimidation of lesbian, gay, and bisexual students for being open and publicly affectionate are so common on college campuses and in the outside world, that there is no point in even listing incidents, as we have done elsewhere in this book.

Exercise for Rating Your Comfort Zones Regarding Lesbian, Gay, and Bisexual Relationships

DIRECTIONS: This exercise is designed for everyone, whether straight, lesbian, gay, or bisexual. Rate the following questions on a scale of 1 to 5, with 1 meaning "extremely uncomfortable," 2 meaning "uncomfortable," 3 meaning "neutral," 4 meaning "comfortable," and 5 meaning "extremely comfortable."

1. Rate your comfort zone when you see images of lesbian, gay, or bisexual relationships in the media (TV programs, online media, movies, books, news reports) when there is no physical affection shown (e.g., the couples depicted are identified as lesbian, gay, or bisexual, but there is no hand-holding, kissing, touching, etc. depicted).

2. Rate your comfort zone when you see images of lesbian, gay, or bisexual relationships in the media and there is some physical affection shown, such as affectionate kissing or hand-holding.

3. Rate your comfort zone when you see images of lesbian, gay, or bisexual relationships in the media and there is strong same-sex erotic/sexual content (R-rated, not pornographic) *of your own gender* depicted, such as sexual scenes on cable TV programs like *The L-Word* or *Queer as Folk* or in movies like *Brokeback Mountain* or *D.E.B.S.*

4. Rate your comfort zone when you see lesbian, gay, or bisexual couples in public whom you do not know personally, and the couples engage in typical displays of public affection, such as hand-holding, light kissing, or affectionate touching.

5. Rate your comfort zone when you are with friends (or acquaintances) involved in lesbian, gay, or bisexual relationships and they engage in displays of public affection in front of you.

6. Rate your comfort zone when you have experienced or might experience a lesbian, gay, or bisexual person of the same sex as you making a compliment (rather than a sexual pass) to you about your appearance ("You look really nice with that new haircut," or "You've really gotten into great shape lately.")

7. Rate your comfort zone when you have experienced (or imagine the possibility of) a lesbian, gay, or bisexual person asking you out on a date (note that this question is not about accepting a date, but about your comfort zone with someone inviting you out on a date).

8. Rate your comfort zone when you have experienced (or imagine the experience of) a lesbian, gay, or bisexual person making a sexual pass at you (note that this question is not about accepting the pass, but about your comfort zone with someone being sexually flirtatious with you).

Because some lesbian, gay, and/or bisexual students might not be "out" and therefore might not want to discuss their responses aloud in class or in groups, this exercise is designed for students to assess their comfort zones in private. Alternatively, students might respond to the questions anonymously, submit their responses to the instructor, and have the instructor tabulate a class average. Note that a class average in the 1 or 2 range or a class average in the 4 or 5 range will not indicate how many students in the class are gay or straight. Some straight students might be so advanced in their acceptance of lesbian, gay, and bisexual relationships that they might be very comfortable with, or even complimented by, a lesbian, gay, or bisexual student making a sexual pass at them, even if they are not interested in an actual sexual encounter with a member of the same sex. At the same time, some lesbian, gay, and/or bisexual students might be very uncomfortable with a sexual pass from a member of the same sex, because they are not ready to explore their sexuality just yet. The point is to assess your comfort zones and advance from that point toward becoming an MRP.

As an MRP, it is your responsibility to come to a point where you not only accept lesbian, gay, and bisexual relationships, but also embrace them. People are either innately interested in same-sex relationships or they're not. Homosexuality is not contagious, so there is no need for people who identify themselves as heterosexuals to be afraid of being in friendly relationships with people who are in intimate same-sex relationships.

Women, Men, and Power

We hope that the previous two sections have made clear how important it is for people striving to become more multiculturally responsible individuals to understand and celebrate intimate relationships that are different from the types of relationships they may be used to seeing in everyday life and in the media. In the previous two sections we discussed societal complications related to alternate types of relationships, but it is also important for MRPs to grasp the importance of unequal power balances within all relationships, whether those relationships are interracial, interethnic, and/or gay/lesbian/bisexual relationships or same race, same ethnicity, and/or heterosexual relationships.

When we talk about unequal power balance in a heterosexual relationship, we are typically talking about the woman being in the position of holding less power than the man. This manifests itself in a number of ways in terms of dating and relationships.

First, unequal power manifests itself in relationships via language. As discussed in Chapter 4, it is still considered acceptable by many to refer to college-age women as "girls," while college-age men are referred to as "men" or "guys" (other than the antiquated term "gals," there is no equivalent non-age-specific term for women in common use). In relationship language, there may be some equality insofar as men and women refer to their partners as "boyfriend" and "girlfriend," but the terminology for the women in the relationship is still often the "girl," while the man in the relationship is the "guy." As a result, the woman is automatically placed into the position of being the less mature and less capable half of the relationship, capitulating to the wants and needs of the man, who is by language placed in the more experienced, more capable position of power.

Another way language lessens a woman's power in dating and relationships is via the use of demeaning, sexist language, which boils women's roles down to just

> ### REFLECTION
>
> If you are a man, imagine being consistently referred to as a "boy" by your professors, coaches, friends, and family. Are you comfortable with this label? How old does it make you feel? If you are a woman, imagine that no one has referred to you as a "girl" since you were 15 years old and that you are now consistently referred to as a "woman." How does this make you feel compared to being referred to as a "girl"?

DEFINITION

Abuse, assault, and rape. There once was a time when there were no such terms as "psychological abuse" or "date rape," but over time, as more and more women (and others) have reported incidents of abuse, assault, and rape, more specific categories have been developed to describe them. *Emotional/psychological abuse* refers to a pattern in which one partner consistently manipulates the other emotionally via ridicule, control, humiliation, or other means, leaving the abused partner feeling worthless and isolated. *Physical abuse* involves using physical violence as opposed to words and behaviors to achieve a similar goal of controlling the victim of the abuse. *Sexual assault* can be either a verbal or physical attack—any form of sexual activity not agreed to by the person being assaulted. Rape is a type of sexual assault, but also under the category of sexual assault are other unwanted sexual advances such as voyeurism, inappropriate groping or touching, exhibitionism, sexualized verbal harassment, and stalking. *Acquaintance rape* is rape committed by someone the victim knows, whether that person is merely an acquaintance or a close friend. *Date rape* is rape committed within a dating situation, in which the rapist assumes that the victim automatically has consented to sexual activity by agreeing to go on a date. Often date rape drugs such as Rohypnol and GHB are involved when a date rape is premeditated.

---

a few categories: helpless creatures ("chick" or "bird"), children ("baby" or "babe"), prostitutes ("bimbo" or "ho"), sexual objects ("stacked" or "hot"), pleasure providers ("sweetie" or "honey"), aggressors ("bitch" and other, even more offensive terms we will not repeat here), or useless/unattractive people ("hag" or "dog"). Women may internalize these terms and feel that they are limited to these roles in a relationship or, in the last case, that they do not deserve to be in a relationship at all.

Second, unequal power manifests itself even more seriously in the emotional/psychological and physical abuse of partners, sexual assault, acquaintance rape, date rape, and rape within relationships. The statistics on these types of abuses of power are difficult to gauge. The most well-documented statistics involve rape. Those statistics reveal that one in four women have been raped in their lifetime, 84% of those women raped knew their attackers, and 57% of those rapes happened on dates (Warshaw, 1994). In other words, 25% of the women you meet in college will be, or already have been, raped in dating situations. Experts agree that the numbers for unreported rapes or attempted rapes are much higher.

REFLECTION

Do you have any friends who have confided in you about being abused, assaulted, or raped? If so, did that friend blame herself or himself or was she or he able to avoid internalizing blame? Why do you think some people might blame themselves for abuse, assault, or rape, when clearly nobody would want these things to happen to them?

Often the aggressors do not comprehend that they have done something wrong, and those attacked feel they brought the aggression upon themselves. Consider the following scenarios, which happen too often on campuses:

- A woman goes out on a date with a friend of a friend. After dinner he drives to a nearby park, overpowers her, and rapes her despite her protests. Alcohol and drugs are not involved. As she is lying in the grass and dirt, he asks if she needs a ride home—and acts like nothing has happened.

- A woman walking across campus late at night is accosted by a group of male students who appear very drunk. One of the male students grabs her on the behind while another gropes her breasts and attempts to kiss her. Although the male students quickly leave the scene and she is not raped, she feels humiliated and violated.

- During a party, drugs are passed around, but nothing with which anyone is unfamiliar. One of the women tries a pill, which her date assures her is just a valium. Half an hour later she is being raped and cannot move. She is aware of everything, but cannot scream. Her friends are 10 feet from her on the patio, but unaware that anything is wrong.

- A woman's boyfriend of 8 months becomes angry and attacks her in her dormitory room. He throws her against her dresser, bruising her, and then picks her up and throws her on the bed. He tears her dress and, because she continues to scream, he takes a pillow and begins to smother her. As she begins to think, "I am going to die," her roommate walks in and stops the situation.

- A woman has been in a relationship with her boyfriend for only a short while, but already she feels powerless. Frequently he orders her around in public, he pulled her by the hair once when he felt she had been engaged too long in a conversation with one of her friends, and he belittles her by commenting on her appearance, sometimes calling her "fat" and sometimes commenting that she has "whorish" taste in clothes. She has thought about breaking up with her boyfriend, but she feels ugly and worthless and wonders if any other men would be interested in her.

It is unfortunate to report that these and other even more outrageous incidents occur every day on college campuses. Notice how all of the incidents involve one individual's power over another. Whether you are male or female, as an MRP it is up to you to understand how an imbalance of power can lead to occurrences of abuse, assault, and rape, not only in dating situations, but also within relationships. Though women are more prone to the consequences of power imbalances than men, men may also be the victims of abuse, assault, and rape in dating and relationships. Typically, the perpetrators are other men. Abuse, assault, and rape are human-wide problems and do not exclusively occur among heterosexuals. In fact, studies indicate that emotional/psychological and physical abuse is as prevalent in same-sex relationships as it is in opposite-sex relationships (National Gay and Lesbian Task Force, 2005). The difference is that there is a distinct lack of support networks in these situations. Shelters for gay men who are being abused or stalked are almost nonexistent. Restraining orders are difficult for lesbian, gay, and bisexual individuals to obtain, and without restraining orders there is no protection. Also, LGB communities tend to be small in most areas, forcing victims of abuse to avoid the LGB community in order to avoid their attackers, which often leaves victims utterly alone.

Gay and bisexual men may be especially vulnerable to sexual assault and rape, because as men, they have not been conditioned to recognize the signs of coercive behavior. Unfortunately, there is also not a great deal of support for males who have been raped, whether gay, bisexual, or straight. Male rape victims often blame themselves for the rape, as a result of societal beliefs that men should be able to protect themselves. Often they do not report being raped and feel unable to talk about the shame they experience after being raped (National Center for Victims of Crime, 1997).

Another group that struggles with abuse, assault, and rape is the transgender community. In fact, transgender individuals are in a particularly vulnerable position in terms of all three forms of violence. Male to female transgender persons are sometimes involved in relationships with men who prefer to perceive of themselves as heterosexual and who may resort to emotional/psychological or physical violence when the fact of their relationship with someone who may not be perceived as "all woman" presents itself. There have also been tragic incidences of violence and even death when a heterosexual man discovers that the woman with whom he had been involved is in fact transgender. Transwomen continue to be vulnerable to sexual assault and rape by men, even if they are particularly feminine in appearance or have already undergone sexual reassignment surgery. This is not, however to say that sexual violence does not exist for female to male transgender people. The most famous example of sexual violence against a female to male transgender person involved Brandon Teena, who was gang raped and later killed by his attackers because, as depicted in the film *Boys Don't Cry*, Brandon left the subordinate female role and assumed male power, something his attackers wished to obliterate.

Exercise for Recognizing Power Imbalances in Intimate Relationships

Some power imbalances in relationships may be easy to recognize by both the people within the intimate relationship and by bystanders, such as situations of rape or physical abuse (though often those who have been raped or physically abused may deny their abuse out of fear). Other power imbalances may not be so easy to spot.

On the following list, place a check mark next to each item that appears to be a case of power imbalance within an intimate relationship, and place an "x" next to each item that may not actually be a case of power imbalance. Sometimes the line between them may be blurry, but practice in learning how to tell the difference will help you become a more aware, more multiculturally responsible individual.

_____ **1.** Diego is a very sloppy dresser, while his girlfriend, Marta, is always immaculately dressed. She says she dresses this way because Diego prefers women who dress nicely.

_____ **2.** Ian gets increasingly anxious about an hour before his partner Mark returns home because of the criticism he is likely to get from Mark.

_____ **3.** Tyrone raises his hand to Ayisha frequently, but he never actually hits her.

_____ **4.** Franklin is always criticizing Katilyn for her horrible taste in music.

_____ **5.** Chaya is always being held so tightly by her boyfriend while they are walking that she looks afraid to take a step without his guidance.

_____ **6.** Susan has threatened to break up with Joy on several occasions because Joy is overweight and does not appear to be doing anything about it.

_____ **7.** Sisa and her husband have not been getting along lately. She feels unattractive and withdrawn.

_____ **8.** Mitch would not dare go out to the movies without checking with his wife, who expects him to check in at least once every hour.

_____ **9.** Paul expects Roger to give him a call at the office once or twice a day to check in.

_____ **10.** Sal uses the term "sweetie" and "baby" to describe his fiancée.

The line may be unclear in some cases, but we believe it is exceedingly clear that the power relationship is unbalanced in items number 2 (there seems to be some emotional abuse contributing to Ian's anxiety), number 3 (the threat of physical abuse is a form of emotional abuse and control), number 5 (Chaya's fear indicates that she is being not only physically but also emotionally controlled), number 6 (threats and humiliation are signs of emotional abuse), and number 8 (constant supervision is a sign of controlling emotional abuse). The other items are more or less benign or, in the case of number 7, an outgrowth of someone's own depression rather than of abuse.

AWARENESS INTO ACTION: ADVOCATING FOR DIVERSE AND SAFE RELATIONSHIPS

As discussed in Chapter 3, we believe that students can learn a great deal from their out-of-class experiences as they do in class. College is not just a place where we take classes, pass tests, write papers, accumulate credits, and graduate. Rather, college is a microcosm of the larger society in which we live. As such, acquiring formal knowledge to prosper in the larger society is part of the picture, but so is learning how to negotiate the world in other ways that are less formalized. One such way of negotiating the world is through establishing various types of relationships with other human beings. Students can learn a great deal through their relationships with others. Book learning and learning from life experiences are essential parts of the learning and living process.

In this chapter there has been a discussion of three important types of relationships that students typically establish and develop in college and continue to establish and develop after graduation. Mentoring relationships are the least potentially controversial, as they are the most formal types of relationships. But it is important to realize how valuable these relationships can be as opportunities to enhance your educational experience.

Friendships are a little more complex because they involve more emotions and complications. This chapter has emphasized the importance not only of developing and maintaining friendships because friends can learn a lot from each other, but also the importance of developing and maintaining friendships with people different from ourselves. Because the college experience fosters diversity and places students in an environment where multi-

> ### QUOTATION
>
> *In the end, we will remember not the words of our enemies, but the silence of our friends.*
>
> MARTIN LUTHER KING JR.
> "The Trumpet of Conscience", 1967

culturalism is much more concentrated, you are strongly encouraged to take advantage of opportunities to appreciate and value other cultures. As an MRP, make every effort you can to celebrate diversity in your own friendships and advocate for the benefits of diverse friendships among others. The lessons you and others learn through diverse friendships in college will carry over into your postgraduation experience and help break down barriers between different racial, ethnic, and cultural groups that exist in the larger society.

Intimate relationships are the most complex kinds of relationships, involving even more emotions and complications than most friendships do. This is highlighted by just how much controversy interracial, interethnic, same-sex, and bisexual intimate relationships still create, and also by the severity of problems that can occur when the balance of power is out of alignment in all types of intimate relationships. We hope this chapter has made it clear that all intimate relationships among consenting adults should be safe and respected. Prejudice against those who are involved in interracial, interethnic, same-sex, and bisexual relationships is unacceptable. In addition, violence within any relationship, whether that relationship is an intimate long-term relationship, a dating relationship, an acquaintance relationship, or an encounter between strangers is also unacceptable.

As an MRP, it is up to you to speak up about and be an advocate for safe, respectful intimate relationships and respect for types of intimate relationships among consenting adults that may be different from those of the majority.

CHAPTER AND PERSONAL REVIEW QUESTIONS

1. What are some of the problems and issues that may get in the way of developing mentor/mentee relationships with professors and other college staff?

2. What is the definition of the term *dyad*, and what are the four types of relationship dyads?

3. What are some of the problems and issues that may get in the way of developing healthy friendships?

4. Now that you have read this chapter, are you motivated to actively seek out friendships with members of racial, ethnic, and cultural groups other than your own? Why or why not?

5. What are some of the problems and issues that people in interracial and interethnic intimate relationships may encounter?

6. How supportive are you of interracial and interethnic intimate relationships? Now that you have read this chapter, are you motivated to move beyond any negative feelings you might have about interracial and interethnic intimate relationships? Please explain.

7. What are some of the problems and issues that people in same-sex and bisexual intimate relationships may encounter?

8. How comfortable are you with same-sex and bisexual intimate relationships? Now that you have read this chapter, are you motivated to move beyond any negative feelings you might have about same-sex and bisexual intimate relationships? Please explain.

9. What are some of the power inequities that may occur in any intimate relationships? What is the difference between emotional/psychological abuse, physical abuse, sexual assault, acquaintance rape, and date rape?

10. Now that you have read this chapter and are aware of the power inequities that may occur within relationships, are you likely to step in and take action when you see such power inequities occurring? Please explain.

REFERENCES

Helms, J. E. (1984). Toward a theoretical explanation of the effects of race on counseling: A Black and White model. *The Counseling Psychologist, 12*(4), 153–165.

National Center for Victims of Crime (1997). Male rape. *National Center for Victims of Crime Website*. Retrieved December 21, 2005, from http://www.ncvc.org/ncvc/main.aspx?dbName=DocumentViewer&DocumentID=32361

National Gay and Lesbian Task Force (2005). Domestic violence. *National Gay and Lesbian Task Force Website*. Retrieved December 21, 205 from http://www.thetaskforce.org/theissues/issue.cfm?issueID=31

Warshaw, R. (1994). *I never called it rape.* New York: HarperPerennial.

▲▲▲
▼▼▼

To Diversity and Beyond: Continuing Your Development as a Multiculturally Responsible Person

BEFORE YOU READ

1. In your personal estimation and through what you have learned in history courses, when do you think things began to take a significant turn for the better for various groups in American society? African Americans? Hispanic/Latino(a) Americans? Asian Americans? Women? Lesbian, gay, and bisexual people? Jewish people? Native Americans? People with disabilities? What groups do you think have not made significant social strides? Why do you think that is the case?

2. What pitfalls have you witnessed or do you think might get in the way of people becoming more multiculturally responsible? How do you think these pitfalls can be avoided?

3. When you finish this book and when this course is over, do you plan to continue to work toward becoming a more multiculturally responsible person? If not, why not? If so, how do you plan to continue your exploration?

INTRODUCTION

Communication and interaction between the majority population and people from racially/ethnically/culturally diverse backgrounds is a relatively new phenomenon in this country. So too is a respectful interaction between men and women as equals. As an example, consider the representation of diverse populations and women on commercial television, which, because it is driven by ratings and advertising to make money, has always aimed to please the greatest number of people with the least amount of risk. Because of its conservative nature, commercial television programming demonstrates just how recently diverse populations and women have gained a voice in our society.

Although *Amos and Andy* featured the first all-Black cast as early as 1951, that program caused a great deal of controversy among African Americans at the time, because it depicted African Americans in a completely stereotypical manner; characters ran the stereotypical gamut, from Amos, an Uncle Tom-like Black conservative, to Andy, his irresponsible, clownish sidekick, to other characters that included a crook, an aggressive mother-in-law, a lazy janitor, and a big-mama character. The only other Black-focused program on television at the time was *Beulah*, featuring an African-American maid working for a White family. It was not until the late 1960s through the 1980s, on programs such as *Julia*, *The Jeffersons*, and *The Cosby Show,* that African Americans began to be represented on television in ways that came from a Black perspective and at least attempted to move away from stereotypical images, even if these shows sometimes courted controversy themselves for various reasons.

Similarly, it was not until the late 1960s and early 1970s that women began to have a voice of their own on American television (that is, they were not depicted as housewives or other caretakers such as maids and nurses) via programs such as *That Girl, The Mary Tyler Moore Show, Maude,* and *Cagney and Lacey*. Jewish characters—at least those clearly identified and allowed to speak for themselves as Jewish—barely appeared on television until various episodes of *All in the Family* dealt with the main character's (Archie Bunker's) anti-Semitism. Only later in the 1970s, on shows such as *Rhoda*, were Jewish characters fully represented in the cast, speaking from their own perspectives. Hispanic characters did not appear on television until the 1970s either, again "introduced" to the American public on episodes of the groundbreaking *All in the Family* and spun off into Hispanic-centered shows such as *Chico and the Man*.

REFLECTION

Have you noticed that nearly all of the television programs mentioned in the preceding paragraphs that broke new ground in terms of multicultural and gender representation were situation comedies? Why do you think that is the case?

The last groups to gain representation have been Asian Americans (to date, there have still been very few programs, save the short-running *All American Girl*, that have consisted of entirely or primarily Asian-American casts), LGBT individuals (such recent shows as *Will and Grace* have centered on gay men, but lesbian, bisexual, and transgender individuals have not had their own voices truly represented on commercial television yet), people with disabilities (who have often been featured in "special" episodes of programs or as members of a larger cast, such as *Joan of Arcadia*, but have yet to be fully represented by any consistently running programs), and such large American populations as Arab Americans, Indian Americans, and those who have lived in America the longest: Native Americans.

> **REFLECTION**
>
> Think of some other, more recent, television programs (commercial television or cable television) that you have watched that are either entirely focused on a racial, ethnic, or cultural minority group, are focused on women, or feature strong central female or diverse characters. In what ways do these programs demonstrate an advancement from the earlier shows, and in what ways are they still multiculturally problematic?

As with our tour of film history in the previous chapter, this brief tour of television history shows that huge strides have been made in the last 30 to 35 years, and these strides reflect the strides made in American society as a whole. Many Americans have watched diverse programming and gained a fuller understanding of and appreciation for people from diverse backgrounds. But there is a large difference between watching and enjoying diverse programming on television and forging real relationships (business relationships, social relationships, friendships, and intimate relationships) with people different from ourselves. So in many ways, we are still in the early stages of a genuinely multicultural society and a number of blunders may still occur that get in the way of our becoming multiculturally responsible persons (MRPs). The first portion of this chapter will address the major pitfalls in the way of multicultural responsibility and how to avoid them to make the road to multicultural responsibility smoother. After these five pitfalls are examined, this chapter (and the book) will conclude with a discussion of ways you can continue multicultural exploration immediately and in the long term after the course in which this book is being used has concluded.

THE FIVE PITFALLS TO MULTICULTURAL RESPONSIBILITY

The five major pitfalls that may hinder the process of developing multicultural responsibility among those who genuinely do want do become MRPs are lack of knowledge, misguided over-dedication, lack of patience, emphasizing shame over accountability, and "positive" stereotyping and countertyping.

Pitfall #1: Lack of Knowledge

The seventeenth-century British poet and essayist Alexander Pope wrote in "An Essay on Criticism," "A little learning is a dangerous thing; drink deep or taste not the Pierian spring; there shallow draughts intoxicate the brain, and drinking largely sobers us again." What Pope meant in these lines was that knowing only a little about a subject is not enough; in fact, a little bit of knowledge may "intoxicate the brain" into feeling a false sense of accomplishment when in fact a little bit of knowledge is only that: a little bit of knowledge. It does not lead to true understanding. To truly understand any subject beyond a superficial level (to be "sober" about a subject, as Pope put it), one must be "drinking largely" from the spring of knowledge. For example, reading one beautifully written and culturally important book by African-American novelist Toni Morrison may give a person a sense of understanding African-American literature and culture, but if it is the only exposure to African-American culture the person ever has, that person will actually know very little about African-American life. The danger is that they will think they do know about the subject and not pursue it further. With regard to becoming a multiculturally responsible participant, a little cursory knowledge about culturally different people, without the depth of lifelong experiences and contact with people different from themselves, can lead people to believe that they have "done their part" or "made an effort" to become MRPs when in fact they have done virtually nothing. The danger in that belief is that racism, ethnocentrism, sexism, homophobia, and other "isms" will persist in our society when most people do not make a concerted effort to combat these problems. As Pope's postulation indicates, MRPs need to immerse themselves in multiculturalism, thereby acquiring a depth of knowledge about people different from themselves rather than skimming the surface of multiculturalism. There is no substitute for long-term personal contact and deep engagement with diversity in the effort to become an MRP.

Ways to increase knowledge and understanding of diversity are limited only to your imagination and creativity. In addition to the action plans we have offered elsewhere in this book for exploring your identity status and expanding your interactions with people from backgrounds other than your own, there are a myriad of books and other media with which you can interact throughout your life to expand your knowledge and understanding of racial/ethnic/cultural/gender history still further. This may sound like a lot of effort, but it does not have to be the equivalent of a lifelong research project. Learning more about others can be much more than a responsibility; it can be a lifetime of enriching experiences. Learning about other cultures can involve reading nonfiction history books, many of which are anything but dry and academic (look at the *New York Times* nonfiction bestseller list; these books are being read by millions because they are interesting and informative). It can involve absorbing diversity while engaged in the pleasurable activities of reading novels, short stories, or poetry, going to see a play, performance art, or poetry slam, watching a movie or television show, listening to a variety of types of music and going to live musical events, or going to an art or cultural exhibit. In addition, increasing your multicultural knowledge and sense of history may involve traveling to other regions within the United States or traveling to other countries and experiencing cultures different from your own firsthand.

Exercise for Increasing Your Knowledge About Diverse Groups and Women's History

DIRECTIONS: This is an out-of-class research exercise. Pick one racial, ethnic, or cultural group (so long as you are not yourself a member of that group) and determine that you are going to focus on that group. You may also focus on women, if you are a man. Complete each of the following steps and write a brief report on what you have learned about your group of choice that you did not already know.

1. Rent one of the DVDs suggested in Chapter 2 that focuses on your group of choice and watch the film with an eye toward gaining understanding of racial, ethnic, cultural, or gender (if your group of choice is women) concerns and issues.

2. Do Web research on your group of choice. Try to find a comprehensive website that outlines your group's history and concerns and also provides links to other websites. When surfing the Web, think critically about choosing an appropriate website. The best websites are .edu or .org websites, which are not profit driven.

3. Interview someone from the group of your choice and ask the person questions about his or her group's history and about the interviewee's family. If your group of choice is women, interview someone who is familiar with women's social history and current women's concerns. If your group of choice is either LGBT people or people with disabilities, focus on group history rather than family history because these individuals are from groups whose families do not necessarily share their cultures.

4. Interview an instructor on campus who is an authority on the history and concerns of your group of choice.

Pitfall #2: Misguided Over-Dedication

Frequently, students will take a course on diversity, read a book, or sit through a training experience and come away elated, feeling inspired to go out and do something to help make the world a better place right away. Such students often become major advocates for oppressed groups and make quick decisions to devote their lives to what they believe is a divine call. You might ask, "So, what's wrong with that? I wish more people were that interested in making the world a better place!" However, diving head first into anything without first acquiring the skills to engage in an action or considering the possible outcomes of one's actions is not always a good thing, either for the individual or for the greater good. For example, take the case of someone who is considering entering the field of social work because he or she is dedicated to making a positive difference in people's lives. The person, who is from an affluent background, volunteers at a soup kitchen for a month and quickly comes to the realization that the facility does not have a large enough food supply to feed everyone who needs to be fed. To compensate, the volunteer goes out to the supermarket daily during the month of volunteering and buys with his or her own money a large quantity of food to make sure everyone is fed. While this may be an extremely heartfelt and noble action on the part of the volunteer, it is ultimately misguided, because once the volunteering stint is over, the homeless will feel a renewed sense of deprivation, the basic problem of food shortages in soup kitchens will not be dealt with at a system-wide level during that month, the increased funding the soup kitchen has been asking for may be ignored by city officials who perceive that there has been no shortage of food, and the volunteer may feel that he or she has made a significant contribution to the homeless population, when in truth he or she has only put a financial Band-Aid on the problem, not contributed any real solutions or honestly grown from the experience.

In terms of multicultural responsibility, consider the case of a student who, after hearing a lecture about the mistreatment of Native Americans throughout American history, dropped out of college to live on a reservation. While this may seem like a noble pursuit, the student did not take the time to research the culture and history of the tribe on a more than superficial level and she rushed into moving to the reservation without considering the impact her decision might have on her future. Almost instantly upon the student's arrival at the reservation, most members of the tribe realized that the student knew very little about their tribal history and customs, and they felt that she condescended to them. In her misguided attempts to reach out as a helper and in her constant focus on the negative historical experiences of the tribe, she never appeared to embrace anything positive about their history and culture and never tried to forge friendships with individual tribe members, seeing them all as a group unified by their oppression rather than as a collection of individuals with a shared history. After a period of trying to practice tolerance of the student, tribe members ended up being exasperated with her and avoided her, leaving her feeling saddened, depressed, and disenchanted. She soon left the reservation and re-enrolled in school, vowed to never get involved in the lives of oppressed people again, and left the tribe members feeling once again patronized by a White person. Clearly her intentions were good, but she might have experienced a more positive outcome if she had taken a more systematic approach. Such an approach might have involved getting to know a few representatives of the tribe who could have taught her more about their ways in preparation for her move to the reservation. In addition, truly getting to know the tribe's culture by reading novels, publications, online newsletters, and viewing documentary films about the lives of Native Americans as a whole and this tribe in particular could have facilitated her learning process. Instead, her over-zealousness (combined with her other pitfall, the lack of knowledge) led to an unproductive, unfulfilling experience that neither helped the tribe nor inspired her to continue making a difference in people's lives, which is a great loss.

The preceding student experience may be an extreme case, but misguided over-dedication can also occur in everyday interactions, so be careful not to jump in too soon as an automatic expert on other people's experiences. Being inspired by a stirring documentary about oppression like *Eyes on the Prize* (the story of the Civil Rights Movement) or *The Times of Harvey Milk* (about the life and murder of gay rights activist Harvey Milk) one day, and talking to members of the groups represented in those films the next day as if you are an expert on those topics will not necessarily ingratiate you to someone who has lived with oppression all of his or her life and has experienced the subject matter of those documentaries firsthand. Having a bad experience when you are trying to make yourself a more aware person may in turn leave you frustrated and dissuade you from further striving to become an MRP. The best advice we can offer is to simply take it step by step; make a realistic action plan for yourself and follow that plan rather than jumping right in when you are not quite ready.

Exercise for Recognizing Misguided Over-Dedication

DIRECTIONS: On the following list, place a check next to each item that seems to be a case of misguided over-dedication and place an "x" next to each item that seems to be appropriate MRP behavior toward getting to know or working with a person from a racial, ethnic, or cultural group other than one's own group.

_____ **1.** Interested in the history of Black players in the early years of integrated baseball, he decided to read a biography of Jackie Robinson.

_____ **2.** Even though she was straight, she decided she would ask a few women out on dates to see what it was like for women to date each other, as she had befriended several lesbian women recently.

_____ **3.** Once he became fully aware of the sexism and homophobia perpetuated by the Greek system in many colleges, he de-pledged his fraternity and vowed never to speak with any of his fraternity brothers ever again.

_____ **4.** She dropped her philosophy minor and switched to Asian-American studies because she was particularly interested in the concerns of Asian Americans and felt that a liberal arts minor focusing on one group would be an initial way to learn about multiculturalism. She maintained her English major.

_____ **5.** Frustrated by the lack of opportunities for recent Hispanic immigrants in America, which she learned about in her sociology course, she neglected all of her courses so that she could take on a full-time job working with the Hispanic immigrant community during her sophomore year.

_____ **6.** Although it was hard work, he decided to start volunteering at a soup kitchen in town five days a week because he cared about the economically disadvantaged.

_____ **7.** Because recent attacks on Arab students had scared him so much, he decided to join the Arab-American student group and run for treasurer of the group, figuring his dedication would override the fact that he was not in fact an Arab American.

_____ **8.** He decided to take an introspective approach to having broken his leg and learn more about persons with disabilities by reading books, talking to students with disabilities, and writing a short story about the experience.

_____ **9.** After she completed her course on multiculturalism, she started a diary in which she recorded her experiences seeking out people from other groups and getting to know them better.

_____ **10.** After reading about the Holocaust, he decided to convert to Judaism, much to the dismay of his Catholic parents.

It is probably readily apparent that items 2, 3, 5, 7, and 10 are examples of over-dedication. Some of these examples may be over the top, but believe it or not, students have gone as far as the students in those examples did to demonstrate their dedication to multiculturalism. What do the examples of appropriate behavior (items 1, 4, 6, 8, and 9) have in common, aside from demonstrating dedication rather than over-dedication?

Pitfall #3: Lack of Patience

In a short poem, American poet Edwin Markham wrote, "He drew a circle that shut me out—/Heretic, a rebel, a thing to flout./But Love and I had the wit to win:/We drew a circle that took him in!" Although most poems are open to multiple interpretations, one fairly obvious interpretation of Markham's poem is that it is about embracing (or pulling into a circle, as Markham puts it) someone who has shut you out, who does not appear to want to be embraced by you. Students striving to become MRPs may at first be surprised that they are not accepted with open arms when they try to reach out to students who are culturally different from them. People striving to become MRPs might be on the receiving end of a comment such as "You've lived a comfortably White existence all of your life and now you want me to be your best friend because you've decided that you like Black people?" or "I've heard you make anti-gay comments before and now you think I owe you something by teaching you how to not be homophobic?", or an MRP may try to help a person with a disability, only to be told sharply that help is not needed.

These are instances when MRPs are just trying to be sensitive, friendly, responsible, nice, or put diversity issues out on the table, so MRPs may be surprised by negative reactions. But it's also important that MRPs keep in mind that many racially, ethnically, and culturally diverse individuals have, through negative experiences, learned to distrust the system and representatives of the system (that is, individuals from the majority race, ethnicity, or culture, or dominant gender). Such individuals may build walls around themselves, protecting themselves from members of the oppressive majority (or in the case of gender, actually the oppressive minority, as women actually outnumber men by 1 to 2%). For this reason, MRPs should understand that just because they have decided to reach out to a member of an oppressed group does not mean automatic acceptance as a saint. In a way, if people expect to be treated like saints for reaching out, are they not exercising privilege? Even if subtly exercising power is not the MRP's intent, it might look that way to someone from an oppressed group.

Consider, for example, the case of a heterosexual student, Doug, whose close friends include a gay man, Dan, and a lesbian woman, Susan. As part of his coming out process and to "clear the air," Dan decides to come out to Doug one day. Doug already had picked up on Dan's subtle hints, but he appreciates the clear gesture on Dan's part. While Susan has not made any attempt to cover up her lesbianism, she has not ever plainly come out to Doug. Doug, feeling he is reaching out to Susan and being fully accepting of her as a friend, asks her why she has never come out to him, to which she responds, "It's not my duty to come out to you." Although it may not have been Doug's intent, he has unconsciously assumed as a member of the privileged group, that it is the duty of the oppressed person to end oppression. Such an experience might be frustrating for Doug, but he needs to not only realize that as a person in the position of power he must consider the viewpoints of others more carefully, and must also understand that he must have patience about being accepted as a multiculturally responsible person. It's not automatic.

While students from majority groups need to have patience with students from oppressed groups who may not automatically embrace their newfound desire to become MRPs, students from oppressed groups are not going to help matters if they are too closed off to accept any outreach at all from others. For example, although in the preceding scenario Susan rightfully remarked that it is not her duty to come out to her friends, she might make an effort to revisit the issue with Doug to clarify her feelings and to remind Doug that she has never tried to hide her sexual orientation from anyone, so why should she think an official coming out moment was necessary? In short, patience works both ways on the path to multicultural responsibility.

Exercise for Assessing Your Level of Patience

As discussed in this section, patience works both ways. Those striving to become MRPs need to realize that people from racial, ethnic, and cultural minorities are not going to instantly applaud a majority group student for his or her efforts, so patience and perseverance are required. On the other hand, those students who are members of racial, ethnic, and cultural minorities need to have patience with those people from majority groups who are honestly trying to become more multiculturally sensitive individuals. With those two sides of the coin in mind, all students who care about multiculturalism should respond to the following questions to assess their level of patience with the sometimes slow process of change.

In the following spaces, place a check mark next to each item that represents a patient response and place an "x" next to each item that represents a level of impatience that may end up impeding multicultural progress.

_____ **1.** Even if equal pay for women takes another 20 years, I am going to keep fighting until that goal is achieved.

_____ **2.** I don't have much time for people who aren't educated in the issues I care about. Too much time is spent training them and not enough getting things done.

_____ **3.** I'm a White, heterosexual male. I know my group is responsible for everything and no one wants to hear from me anyway, so I'm going to just hang back and let others make the world a better place.

_____ **4.** When I meet a first-year student who is full of stereotypes about everybody, I make a point of trying to befriend that person rather than writing her or him off immediately.

_____ **5.** Homophobes are homophobes and there's no changing that.

_____ **6.** I came to this college knowing that it was relatively conservative, but it's a great institution, so I think it's worth working within and making gradual changes.

_____ **7.** Change has come from within the most unexpected places on campus, so I think people should be given a chance to make their contribution to the overall multicultural climate on campus, even if some factions are slow about it.

_____ **8.** We need to close the fraternities and sororities now. These are racist, sexist, homophobic institutions and nothing's going to change that.

_____ **9.** I was initially displeased with the addition of transgender people to the lesbian, gay, and bisexual movement (it used to be LGB, not LBGT), because it makes our point even harder to get across to a sometimes confused mainstream, but if lesbian, gay, and bisexual people don't reach out to help transgender people move forward, who will?

_____ **10.** Old activists hold back student movements towards multiculturalism. They are too stuck in their outdated views to really help.

As usual with these types of exercises, sometimes the lines are fuzzy, but in our opinion, items 1, 4, 6, 7, and 9 represent appropriate patience. Although some of the sentiments expressed in items 2, 3, 5, 8, and 10 represent a desire to more forward quickly and finally get to a place where racism, sexism, homophobia, etc. no longer exist, the way to do that is to learn from others rather than discount them (or ourselves) based on "newbie" or "veteran" status, or perceptions of them being beyond hope or too much trouble.

Pitfall #4: Emphasizing Shame Rather Than Accountability

In the process of becoming multiculturally responsible, students should learn how to differentiate between accountability and shame. Failure to understand the difference between the two and emphasizing shame over accountability poses a tremendous threat to empathic understanding and renders people powerless to form positive multicultural connections. For example, consider the case of a student who comes from a White, very privileged background, whose family history goes back to the American Colonial era and involved the ownership of slaves (therefore the family profited from the exploitation of human beings), and whose family continues to live in a primarily White neighborhood in which racist comments are often heard. The student herself may have always empathized with people from all types of backgrounds, or she may have become close with someone from a different race at some point in her life, which caused her to question the legacy of racism that exists in her family, or a family member or schoolteacher may have opened her eyes about the wrongs of racism and other forms of oppression at some point in her life. Regardless of how she came to realize that she has been privileged as a White person all her life, she has two choices as to how she is going to react to that understanding. She can either choose to be ashamed of her family history and not be able to look her African-American fellow students in the face, or she can take accountability for her own racial privilege and make positive strides against racism and oppression in her personal life, or in her activities, or both. Denying the legacy of racism in America's past and in her own family would not be a viable option, because that would be simply lying to herself and to others. However, living in shame would not be a viable option either, as no positive outcomes can result from lack of action.

> **DEFINITION**
>
> *Accountability* and *Shame. Accountability* is the acceptance of responsibility for an action or behavior that is considered wrong, or the acknowledgement of one's part in something wrong. *Shame* is a strong emotional reaction caused by guilt, embarrassment, or disgrace. Individuals who experience shame believe that they are intrinsically bad or worthless individuals, whereas individuals who accept accountability are able to move forward.

On the opposite side of the coin, emphasizing shame over accountability can be a pitfall toward multicultural responsibility when people from diverse, oppressed backgrounds hold shame over the heads of people from majority or privileged backgrounds who are striving to become MRPs. While this is not to say that members of oppressed groups should not hold people from majority groups accountable for oppression (either directly or indirectly by privilege), it is to say that nothing can be accomplished when multicultural responsibility is prevented from developing. If an African-American heterosexual student and a White gay student are to work together to help reduce oppression in the world, they will first need to learn how to avoid shaming each other as the root causes of racism and heterosexism.

Exercise for Recognizing the Difference Between Accountability and Shame

DIRECTIONS: Mark with a check mark the following items that represent accountability and mark with an "x" those items that represent shame. Recognizing the difference will help both people from the majority groups and those from minority groups make a clear distinction that will allow them to not get stuck in what might be called the "shame trap."

_____ **1.** I have a hard time dealing with Jewish people, knowing that my father made all of those anti-Semitic comments at the dinner table when we were growing up.

_____ **2.** I've told a lot of homophobic jokes in my time, but since my sister came out as a lesbian I'm trying to make an effort to be a better person.

_____ **3.** I know people don't like to feel guilty about things they didn't do personally, but I think anyone who isn't Native American should accept the fact that they ultimately benefit from previous generations' exploitation of the Native Americans.

_____ **4.** White people are essentially racist and there's nothing that can be done about it.

_____ **5.** My ancestors had to deal with anti-Irish sentiments when they first arrived in New York at the turn of the century, but I'm still White, so I can't ignore the fact that racism is part of my legacy.

_____ **6.** I get so nervous when I think Black people are going to confront me about racism that I'm afraid I'm going to blurt out something racist just out of nervous confusion.

_____ **7.** I don't feel that I can ever forgive men for their basic disregard for women, which I experience every day.

_____ **8.** Men need to realize that they still hold power in our society and stop pretending that women have caught up.

Items 1, 4, 6, and 7 all have a commonality: change is not seen as an option because the speakers either feel so ashamed or are so determined not to forgive that they shame others. These people will not be able to interact with others to move past shame and make genuine progress. The speakers in items 2, 3, 5, and 8 all realize that even if they are not directly responsible for inequities in society, nothing is going to change if they do not take accountability for their privileges and work with others to facilitate change.

Pitfall #5: "Positive" Stereotypes and Countertypes

Negative stereotypes are not the only types of stereotypes—they are just the most egregious types of stereotypes, because they are so obviously designed to dehumanize members of racial/ethnic/cultural minority groups and women by boiling their entire existence down into just a few ugly traits. Negative stereotypes once common in the media, such as the African-American mammy, the swishing homosexual, or the cheap Jewish person are rarely depicted in the media anymore, and people who employ negative stereotypes in the workplace today are liable to be quickly corrected, if not immediately scheduled for diversity training.

"Positive" stereotypes (e.g., stereotyping all Black men as athletic, all Black women as strong, all Asian-Americans as intelligent, all Hispanic/Latino(a) Americans as morally centered, all gay men as artistically talented, all lesbian women as socially conscious, all Jews as financially adept, all women as nurturing, etc.) do not appear to be hurtfully offensive, but they nonetheless serve to limit the realm of human potential of people who happen to be part of larger groups.

Another type of stereotype, which is perhaps the least overtly offensive is the countertype. The problem with countertypes, however, is that they are often perceived by persons striving to become MRPs as complimentary, yet stereotypes are still stereotypes. No matter how nice they may look, they still put people into boxes.

Positive stereotypes and countertypes are some of the most difficult pitfalls to overcome on the way to multicultural responsibility because these images are everywhere we look. In terms of positive stereotypes, there may be a large number of gay men involved

> **DEFINITION**
>
> *Countertype.* A *countertype* is a form of stereotype designed to counter a familiar negative stereotype, but it is still a stereotype and therefore does not represent the complexity of people from different groups. Examples include "Buppies" (Black urban professionals, countering the negative stereotype of African Americans as unemployed, underemployed, or lazy), "kickass" women (women who fight as hard as men, countering the stereotype of women as passive and nurturing), "lipstick lesbians" (lesbians who dress stylishly and use cosmetics, countering the stereotype of the unfeminine lesbian), and "butch" gay men (gay men who like sports and beer, countering the stereotype of the effeminate gay man).

in the fashion and beauty industries and these men may be celebrated on television shows such as *Queer Eye for the Straight Guy* and *Project Runway*, but when these are among the very few images of gay men on television, such positive stereotypes limit the ability of gay men to see themselves as anything different from these stereotypes and keep others from viewing gay men as anything much more than superficial. In terms of countertyping, there are many Hispanic Americans finding great success in business, law, medicine, and other high-income careers, but if the only images anyone sees of Hispanic Americans on television are those involving affluence and yuppiedom (i.e. Young Urban Professional), then the range of Hispanic-American experience becomes a limited one, one which renders the large non-affluent Hispanic-American population invisible and which quietly invalidates Hispanic Americans who have accents, do not dress in "proper" (i.e. nonethnic) attire, and have not given up their heritage in favor of a "professional" attitude. MRPs should be aware that stereotypes are stereotypes, no matter how seemingly complimentary or contrary to the old negative stereotypes they seem to be. Like their uglier predecessors, these new stereotypes do not encourage people to learn about diversity; rather these new stereotypes tend to shut down conversation.

Exercise for Recognizing "Positive" Stereotypes and Countertypes

DIRECTIONS: To gain a deeper understanding of some of the positive stereotypes and countertypes we see in the media and may perpetuate ourselves, make a list of both positive stereotypes and countertypes next to each of the following groups. Because this is a brainstorming activity, more responses will be generated by completing this exercise as a group.

Women:

_____

People from specific countries of the world/Ethnic groups in America (e.g., Brazilians/Brazilian Americans, Swedish/Swedish Americans):

_____

Africans/African Americans/Black people:

_____

Europeans/European Americans/White people:

_____

Asians/Asian Americans:

_____

Hispanics/Hispanic Americans:

_____

Native Americans:

_____

LGBT people:

_____

Arabs/Arab Americans:

_____

Indians/Indian Americans:

_____

Economically disadvantaged people:

_____

Middle-class people:

_____

Wealthy people:

_____

People with disabilities (physical or mental):

_____

Protestants:

_____

Catholics:

_____

Jewish people:

_____

Muslims:

_____

People of other religious affiliations (Hindi, Buddhist, Jehovah's Witness, Seventh Day Adventist, etc.):

_____

AWARENESS INTO ACTION: CONTINUING YOUR EXPLORATION AS AN MRP

Throughout this book, you have learned a great deal about multicultural responsibility and about becoming a multiculturally responsible participant. You have been encouraged to become aware of and examine your own attitudes and feelings in situations where diversity is involved. You have been encouraged to understand and respect the worldviews of people different from yourself. You have also been invited to become keenly aware of diversity in all aspects of campus life by exploring your racial/ethnic/cultural identity status, becoming aware of privilege, understanding the variables students experience both in and out of the classroom, exploring the factors that influence relationships, and understanding the pitfalls that might get in the way of multicultural responsibility. Now let's give someone who disagrees with our fundamental philosophy—that multicultural responsibility is not only something that should be discussed, but something that should be actively fought for—a chance to disagree.

A Voice of Dissent

Given what you have learned from this book, we would like you to respond to a commentary written by a student who is resistant to the idea of multicultural responsibility on campus. Please read the following excerpt, in which the anonymous student critiques various aspects of his or her college's diversity mission statement. After you have read the excerpt, identify and discuss the comments with which you agree and those with which you disagree. If you were presented with an opportunity to debate the anonymous writer, what key points would you use to support your position?

> However, the more glaring flaw of this aspect of [our mission statement] is its emphasis on artificially forcing the makeup of the faculty and student body to be something that it is not. The first goal of the "Diversify and Globalize" tenet states that "recruitment activities must focus on students and their parents in targeted school districts and community colleges thorough strategically located outreach centers and through utilizing students and faculty of diverse backgrounds in recruiting activities." Clearly, this goal is intended to actively recruit students who have a certain set of characteristics over other students. I would have no problem with such a goal, were the characteristic in question intelligence, or work ethic, or aptitude for a particular subject matter. This is not the case, however. [This college] is seeking to recruit students and faculty who are of a specific ethnic or racial background, at the expense of others. This is racism. Consider if the situation was reversed, and [this college] sought to target only wealthy White students from rural school districts. This would be wrong, and no court in the land would uphold such activity. Why, then, is it considered not only acceptable, but also obligatory to reverse-discriminate?

Consider an alternative approach. Let's stop talking about race altogether. Let's stop caring what the outside world says about our campus being too White or too Black or too green or whatever. We don't let public criticism of our yell leaders force us to form a cheerleading squad. Why should this debate be any different? Let's make sure we offer a demanding curriculum, which educates any person who cares to attend this institution. Let's conduct research that pushes the limits of our current understanding of the world. This way, the best students and the best faculty in the nation and in the world will be proud to cite an affiliation with [our college]. Any student, of any race, who graduates with a degree from this school, will be able to effectively compete in the business world. We can offer no better incentive to any individual to attend this university than that.

Finally, let me cite one more aspect of [our diversity plan] with which I fundamentally disagree. It states, "To position our students to live and compete in a global society, [this University] must produce graduates who are not only academically prepared, but who have the capacity to understand other cultures and to live and work outside their own cultural framework." This is true. However, forcing a multicultural student body can never achieve this goal. For example, I remember my high school, which had an extremely "diverse" campus. Over 50% of the student body consisted of minority students. Still, most had no idea of how to appropriately interact with each other. During class meetings, I noticed how consistently the students chose to sit only with members of their own race. The de facto segregation was striking. You see, just because multiple races of students attend a single campus does not mean that they will be forced to understand each other's cultures. Only individual volition can transcend cultural differences. No one, not a school, nor a leader, nor any government institution, can force a person, against his will, to accept another culture if he is unwilling to do so.

In conclusion, I believe that the emphasis on multiculturalism that is so prevalent on our campus these days is nothing more than an attempt to achieve a superficial appearance of acceptance, so that we will be able to satisfy the demands of our "politically correct" culture.... Advocates of multiculturalism on campus, whether intentionally or not, are proclaiming that the measure of a man is not the content of his character, but the color of his skin. And I, for one, do not intend to stand by quietly and watch this university violate its honorable heritage by continuing to pursue such a racist mentality.

The student's comments are convincing, well written, and thought provoking. However, one of the student's central arguments is that if we do not pay attention to race (or by implication, ethnicity or culture), these issues will eventually disappear. There are going to be times when people think this way—good people with good intentions. Well-written articles will cause people to pause and wonder if actively pursuing diversity is a worthwhile endeavor. However, we would like to state our case, as we have elsewhere in the book, that racism, ethnocentrism, sexism, homophobia, classism, ageism, and the many other "isms" that still exist in our society, are not going to go away simply by ignoring them. We would like to argue that ignoring these issues (or being powerless to confront them) is what allowed them to grow in the first place. The student argues that no court in the land would uphold a policy that only allowed for the recruitment of White students. But is this not exactly the policy that used to exist on most college campuses in the United States prior to the 1960s? Were it not for forced desegregation of elementary schools, high schools, and colleges set in motion by the landmark *Brown vs. Board of Education* Supreme Court decision in the 1950s, Black and other culturally diverse students would not be sitting in college classrooms across America today.

Another point the student makes is that placing diverse people together does not necessarily improve diversity on campus. Rather, it just creates an artificial sense of diversity, when in fact students will still gravitate to other students like them. Although this is true, the student uses this as an argument against recruitment of minority students. However, recruitment and retention of minority and nontraditional students provides the opportunity to have these diversity discussions, and without those opportunities, nothing will change. Personal contact and difficult discussions will improve diversity issues. In addition, let's not forget our lengthy conversation about privilege. In a perfect world, all students would have the same advantages and would all be on an equal playing field during the college application process. Unfortunately, this is not a realistic expectation, even in this day and age. Minority students, particularly African-American and Hispanic-American students, are still overwhelmingly schooled in poverty-stricken, under-funded school districts and, despite equal aptitude, simply are not as well prepared for college entrance as students from mostly White, privileged school districts. Therefore, the student makes a mistake in assuming that ignoring race will naturally attract diverse students.

Lastly, the student argues that, "Only individual volition can transcend cultural differences. No one, not a school, nor a leader, nor any government institution, can force a person, against his will, to accept another culture if he is unwilling to do so." On the surface, this is true, but the goal of multicultural education is not to force anyone's hand. We certainly hope that the message you have gotten out of this book is not that this is a book designed for a course in Brainwashing 101. Rather, it is hoped that multicultural education, whether that be in the context of a specific course on multiculturalism, as a by-product of a course in a specific discipline (such as history, literature, or political science), or outside of the classroom, will open the eyes of students to broader ways of thinking, or "thinking outside of the box." Whether they choose to embrace broader ways of thinking or not is up to students themselves. But is that not what education on the whole is all about: broadening one's thinking? What would some of the world's greatest artists, law makers, businesspeople, speakers, writers, historians, and others have become if they had never sought to expand their horizons and measure alternative points of view against their own? By the same token, since we are talking essentially about the discipline of sociology in this book, where would our society be now if individuals had never questioned their points of view and adjusted them to the greater good? It is our strong opinion, and that of most historians, that if no one ever questioned that social status quo (in short, if no one ever attempted multicultural exploration) the world would still be living in ancient times, times when religious differences were stamped out with violence, women were unquestioningly subservient to men, slave ownership was a fact of life, and those perceived as outsiders were summarily executed.

Of course those times are long past and seem almost mythical to us today, but we did not get to where we are today by unwaveringly staying the course. Considering that most world societies are now closer to harmony than ever before, albeit with many problems that still persist, is talking about diversity, taking a course in the topic, and reaching out to help even the playing field really that much of a sacrifice?

Continuing the Conversation

One way to completely avoid blunders related to multiculturalism is to never communicate or interact with people from groups other than your own. Since that is not a realistic goal for getting through life in our increasingly multicultural and globalized world, people are encouraged to get involved regularly with people who are different from themselves. Contact coupled with genuine caring, respect, and sensitivity can be achieved through the following general guidelines:

1. **Self-Awareness:** Students are encouraged to become aware of their identity development statuses and work toward moving ahead to the next level. Students who have achieved the highest levels of identity development should reach out and help others who have not advanced to the highest level.

2. **Awareness of Attitudes Toward Others:** Students are encouraged to become more aware of their true attitudes and feelings toward the racially, ethnically, and culturally different, and should be actively engaged in an ongoing process of changing those attitudes and feelings that are negative.

3. **Awareness of Privilege:** Students are encouraged to become aware of the various types of privilege that exist in our society and work to not only overcome privilege in general but also to reject their own privileges for the sake of the greater good.

4. **Awareness of Others' Differences:** Students are encouraged to work toward greater empathy of those different from themselves by recognizing that not all students experience the classroom situation, out-of-class campus life, and campus relationships in the same way.

5. Acquisition of Knowledge: Students are encouraged to become involved in an ongoing process of acquiring knowledge and insight about the worldviews of diverse individuals through a wide variety of media including books, movies, and above all, personal contact with individuals from different groups.

6. Action: Students are encouraged to practice a wide range of culturally sensitive communication strategies and should actively seek out opportunities to expand their interactions with those who are different from themselves, so long as the potential pitfalls have first been examined.

As we have indicated throughout this book, the process of becoming multiculturally responsible is ongoing. It does not end with graduation. Issues regarding diversity will continue to affect you throughout your life: in your personal life, in your community, at work, and at a governmental level. Eventually the term *minority* will be replaced, because, based on United States population projections, White people will become the minority. Every day the United States and the world are changing. Within the United States, one major change is toward diverse representation in all facets of life. On the global scale, the world is moving in a direction (due in a large part to the proliferation of the Internet) in which countries are no longer as isolated and self-contained as they once were—international interaction is now the rule rather than the exception. We encourage each individual to recognize and embrace these proposed changes as tools for connecting and interacting with people with differences, in a sincere effort to make the world a better place to live.

QUOTATION

I swear never to be silent whenever and wherever human lives endure suffering and humiliation. We must always take sides... When human dignity is in jeopardy, that place, at that moment, must become the center of the universe.

ELIE WIESEL
Nobel Peace Prize acceptance speech, December 10, 1986

Now that you have read this book, what is your next step toward becoming multiculturally responsible?

CHAPTER AND PERSONAL REVIEW QUESTIONS

1. What are the five pitfalls to multicultural responsibility?

2. In what ways is lack of knowledge a pitfall to multicultural responsibility and in what ways can it be overcome?

3. In what ways is misguided over-dedication a pitfall to multicultural responsibility and in what ways can it be overcome?

4. In what ways is lack of patience a pitfall to multicultural responsibility and in what ways can it be overcome?

5. In what ways is the emphasis of shame over accountability a pitfall to multicultural responsibility and in what ways can it be overcome?

6. What is the definition of a "positive" stereotype? What is the definition of a countertype?

7. In what ways are "positive" stereotypes and countertypes pitfalls to multicultural responsibility and in what ways can they be avoided?

8. What are the six guidelines to follow for continued pursuit of multicultural responsibility? Are you motivated to follow these guidelines throughout college and beyond?

Index